SEEKING
SLOW

RECLAIM MOMENTS OF
CALM IN YOUR DAY

Melanie Barnes
creator of Geoffrey and Grace

ROCK
POINT

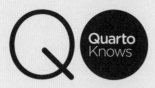

Inspiring | Educating | Creating | Entertaining

Brimming with creative inspiration, how-to projects, and useful information to enrich your everyday life, Quarto Knows is a favorite destination for those pursuing their interests and passions. Visit our site and dig deeper with our books into your area of interest: Quarto Creates, Quarto Cooks, Quarto Homes, Quarto Lives, Quarto Drives, Quarto Explores, Quarto Gifts, or Quarto Kids.

Text and Photography © 2019 by Melanie Barnes

First published in 2019 by Rock Point, an imprint of The Quarto Group, 142 West 36th Street, 4th Floor, New York, NY 10018, USA T (212) 779-4972   F (212) 779-6058 www.QuartoKnows.com

Rock Point titles are also available at discount for retail, wholesale, promotional and bulk purchase. For details, contact the Special Sales Manager by email at specialsales@ quarto.com or by mail at The Quarto Group, Attn: Special Sales Manager, 100 Cummings Center Suite, 265D, Beverly, MA 01915, USA.

Library of Congress Control Number: 2019943789

10 9 8 7 6 5 4 3

ISBN: 978-1-63106-630-6

Group Publisher: Rage Kindelsperger
Creative Director: Laura Drew
Managing Editor: Cara Donaldson
Senior Editor: Erin Canning
Art Director: Cindy Samargia Laun
Cover Design: Evelin Kasikov
Page Design: Laura Shaw Design

Printed in China

For all the seekers of slow who believe that there is a better way to live.

To my family, who fill my life with joy and inspire me to live slowly,
be present, and make the most of our time together.

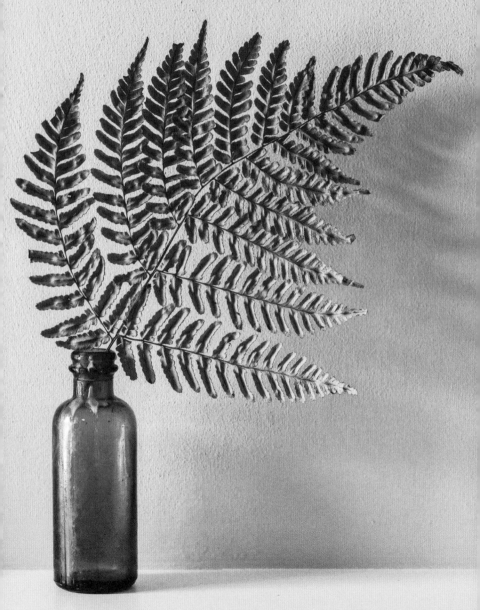

CONTENTS

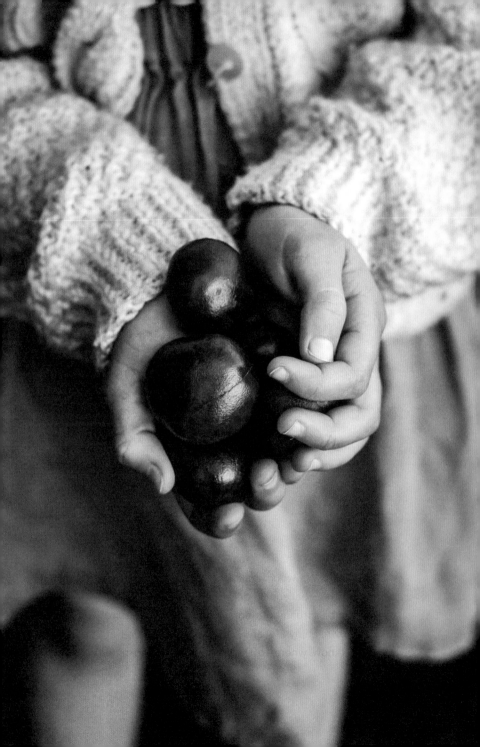

PREFACE

It was not long after my daughter was born that we started to explore slow living. It all started with a gradual realization that time is a precious commodity that we cannot get back. Becoming a mother highlighted to me how fleeting time can be as I watched how quickly our baby was growing into a little girl. I didn't want to miss a minute of it because I was rushing through life too busy or too stressed. I wanted to be as present as possible and soak in her childhood and every little detail—the fun and the challenging.

Through the early years of our daughter's life, I found that my perspective on many things altered. What was once important didn't seem so important anymore, and I discovered new priorities. In response to these changes, we began to adapt the way we approached life as a family. We began to think about what was essential and what could be simplified. On examining my motivation for slowing life down, I knew I wanted to be as intentional and present with my time as possible; however, I also realized that I needed to prioritize my and my family's well-being, and that slow living would facilitate this.

During this time, I had a recurring conversation with many people. We would talk about our difficulties in balancing the challenges of life: work, parenthood, paying the bills, running a home, etc., with this desire to slow down, enjoy life, and generally feel better. But we didn't know where to start or how to make time to do so. Slowing down and prioritizing our well-being seemed to be an unfamiliar concept to many of us.

When I looked a little closer, I realized that I had in many ways always been a proponent for slow living—we all have things we do so naturally that we never question them or consider that they might be unique. From a young age, I remember wanting to feel connected to my body. I thought that if I understood my body and all its facets, I would therefore understand myself. Learning to appreciate and listen to my body has naturally always allowed me to be guided by my well-being. I assumed everyone approached life this way and that being "in your body" and listening to your body was instinctual to all of us. As I entered further into adulthood, I realized that this was not the case and that many people live their whole lives without being truly connected to their bodies.

Studying dance and movement, and then yoga, meditation, and holistic therapies later in my life, meant that I had the opportunity to deeply explore the connection to myself: how my body moves, what its limits are, the body-mind connection, and how to restore and nurture myself. Spending time learning about the human body and mind in this way naturally changed the context of how I viewed myself, and an increase in the awareness of my general well-being automatically followed suit.

Having spent fifteen months exploring my craft as a dancer in New York City and taking as many dance, movement, and yoga classes as possible, I had stretched my body to its limits. I was as connected to my physical body as I was ever going to be, but I started to think that perhaps there were other elements that were missing. On returning to the UK, I went through a lengthy spell of feeling unwell, and went back and forth to the doctor. Eventually, there was a vague diagnosis of irritable bowel syndrome, and in terms of treatment, little guidance and help were offered, which encouraged me to explore changing my diet and how I could better support my body holistically. After about six months of dietary changes and altering some of my habits and routines, I started to feel well again. I could see that the changes I had made to my lifestyle were having a positive impact.

Approaching life holistically allowed me to think about my body and my well-being in a more complete way. I realized how important it was to consider the whole picture when making choices and decisions about myself and my loved ones. As well as taking into account my physical health, holistic living encouraged me to look at my mental and emotional health and consider the impact of stress and anxiety. Realizing that everything is intimately interconnected changes how we respond to looking after ourselves.

My experience had taught me that it was possible to feel better by simply altering aspects of my lifestyle. I wanted others to be able to benefit in the same way, so I decided to look further into the things that had improved my well-being. I studied yoga, yoga philosophy, and meditation before becoming a Kundalini yoga teacher and massage therapist. On many occasions, I had to encourage myself to embrace unconventional philosophies when seeking well-being ideas and inspiration, realizing that we must try something and experience it before passing judgment on whether it can be of any benefit to us.

Teaching was incredibly rewarding, as I would see a noticeable shift in people in the space of just a class. They would come in looking tired or frazzled and leave breathing a little deeper and looking more relaxed. I spent nearly all my twenties and early thirties studying or teaching yoga, movement, and meditation, yet in my early thirties, something happened that created a disconnect within myself. Everything that I had learned and had been practicing, gradually began to fall away as I slipped further into a state of depression and isolated myself more and more.

Anyone who has had difficulties in becoming a parent and with infertility will know what a painful and lonely time it can be. Month after month went by without a positive result, and then months turned into years, and still we had no answers. I struggled to cope with the constant disappointment and the uncertainty of it all. I felt let down by the fact that my body didn't seem to be able to do what I wanted the most. I had spent the last fifteen years learning to be connected to my body and consider my well-being, yet it didn't seem to make a difference when it came to wanting to become a mother. After a difficult three and half years, I had just come to terms with the fact that we probably wouldn't be able to have any children, when a few months later we became pregnant.

After our daughter was born, that sense of time being precious was no doubt amplified by the fact that it took us such a long time to conceive. The early years of our daughter's life inspired my first steps into slow living, and I began sharing my thoughts about motherhood and simplifying our lives on Instagram and on my blog, Geoffrey and Grace. Through reading, writing, and talking about my experiences, I realized that many others were also feeling this desire to slow down and simplify, in order to connect with the important things in life. I thought about the things we were doing that were helping our family slow down and feel good, and wanted to share them. Gradually, through conversation with friends and family, I remembered how I had always been drawn to think about my body and prioritize my well-being. Perhaps now I could help others slow down and feel more connected to their bodies in the same way.

Geoffrey and Grace initially started as a creative project purely for pleasure, but it has now grown from a blog to guiding and impacting all parts of my life—from becoming my full-time job to influencing our lifestyle choices as a family.

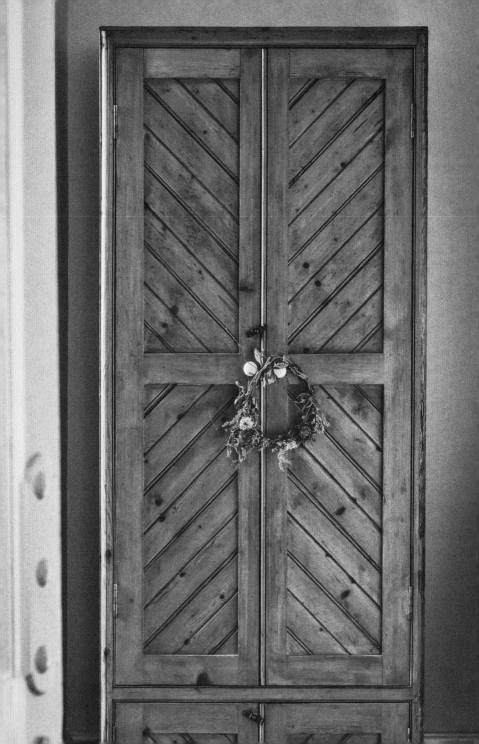

Slow Living

AN INTRODUCTION

....

What would happen if we lived our lives at a slower pace? If we occasionally paused for thought, simplified our lifestyles, and created space for moments of stillness, perhaps we would also find more joy and happiness. We all know how easy it is to get swept away with a busy day; time can pass in a bit of a blur and we often don't feel like we were there for any of it. In order to be the happiest and healthiest we can be, it is necessary to look at slowing down and reconnecting to ourselves. Living slowly and simply is the perfect antidote to the hustle and bustle of twenty-first-century life.

WHAT IT MEANS TO LIVE
A SLOW AND SIMPLE LIFE

Simple living is not a new concept—people have been practicing it for centuries—and the term "slow living" as we know it today is becoming increasingly popular. Used to describe a lifestyle that encourages a slower rhythm and values a mindful approach, slow living isn't about doing everything slowly. It is about intentionally doing things and being present for each part of our day. By choosing quality over quantity, we gain more opportunity to savor the simple pleasures and experience those moments wholeheartedly.

An alternative approach to living in the fast lane started with the Slow Food movement in the 1980s. When a famous fast food chain wanted to open a branch near the Spanish Steps in Rome, residents, politicians, and officials opposed the idea. This single event prompted Carlo Petrini to found the Slow Food movement as an alternative to fast food. Its aim: to defend traditions, celebrate the pleasure of food, and highlight the connection between where our food comes from and how it ends up on our plates. Over the last thirty years, the ideas behind the Slow Food movement have crept into mainstream culture and expanded into other areas of our lives. With working weeks seeming longer, schedules more rigorous, and people appearing busier than ever before, slow living is becoming an essential practice for our well-being.

It is not surprising that we are looking for ways to simplify and slow down. Many of us are living beyond our means, in terms of energy, resources, and time—we have come to expect a lot from our bodies and our lifestyles. Often, we are juggling things or multitasking in the quest to "have it all" or "do it all." There will always be more tasks to do, more emails to answer, more work to catch up on. Add to this the brilliance of technology and we can now do these things at any time of the day, even when we would have previously been resting or doing nothing. This can leave us with the expectation that we must use our time more efficiently. The pressure that comes hand in hand with feeling busy means we often hurry through our days, which results in us being less productive with our time and missing out on life's wonderful moments.

Most of us instinctively know there is a better way to live our lives than being hustled along an endless track of "to-do lists." Destination living, where we are fixed solely on a specific end point or result, means we are more likely to miss out on enjoying the small and simple experiences along the way. Still, slowing down can seem challenging. So, how do we realistically slow down and navigate the misconceptions about who slow living is suitable for?

REALISTIC SLOW LIVING

Slow living is possible for everyone. The art of slow living is not in how much "free time" you have, but how intentional you are with that time. There are many facets to slow living that can be applied practically to anyone's lifestyle—from slow food and slow fashion to slow travel and slow parenting.

By examining our attitude to time, we can alter how we approach individual tasks and how we schedule our week. By analyzing our purpose and prioritizing, we can understand what is motivating us and fill our days accordingly. Through slowing our homes and simplifying our belongings, we can begin to create space for more rest and play. By looking to nature and the seasons for inspiration, we can see how living seasonally can naturally shape and slow down our rhythms and routines.

Once we start to live slowly, we automatically begin to increase our awareness of our general well-being. We need to remember that time nurturing and tending to ourselves isn't a luxury, but is, in fact, essential, and that we must reconnect and learn to listen to our bodies in order to truly slow down. We don't need a lot of time; just ten minutes daily can go a long way to support our health and happiness.

By mindfully approaching everyday tasks, we can begin to slow down our minds and thoughts. In this book, I will be encouraging you to think deeply about the choices you make across all areas of your life. It is important to invest some time and energy to think about how you spend your days, what you spend your money on, what leisure activities you choose to do, and what things you surround yourself with. All of this filters into effect how slowly we are able to live our lives, and how lightly we are able to tread on this earth.

We often equate happiness with the big moments in life, but there is a lot of joy to be found in the simple things. Let's learn to cherish those small moments, and refocus what it means to be happy—it is not about trying to have it all, but about learning to be content with what we have, and that less can indeed be more.

REFLECTING ON THE PAST

Generations before us managed to live slowly and simply, in part because the way people used to live facilitated a slower and simpler existence, though often it was out of necessity through times of austerity, and living could be hard. My grandparents grew their own vegetables because of food rations; they mended stuff because they didn't have the money to throw things away and replace them with something new. Simple things, such as a trip to the cinema or gathering around the telly to watch a TV show as it first aired, were hotly anticipated and felt like a treat. Generally, there were a lot fewer distractions, so it was easier to go at a slower pace and find time to spend with family. Shops were often closed on Sundays; therefore, enjoying long family lunches, playing games, spending time in nature, and even being bored were normal pastimes.

There were also fewer choices about how to spend leisure time and less information readily available to everyone. People had to seek out their own entertainment and fun, so they often invested more time in hobbies. Though more time was spent on doing household chores—washing everything by hand, mending clothes, cooking from scratch—that have since been replaced by "easier" time-saving alternatives, we still feel as if there aren't enough hours in the day.

While in one respect it is wonderful to have so much choice and flexibility with what we can do and when, it is important that we are mindful about how we choose to spend our free time, and that we invest our energy in activities that bring us joy and enhance our well-being. Especially where self-esteem and self-worth are concerned, perhaps, in some ways, our ancestors had the right idea. It is probably healthier to spend our time

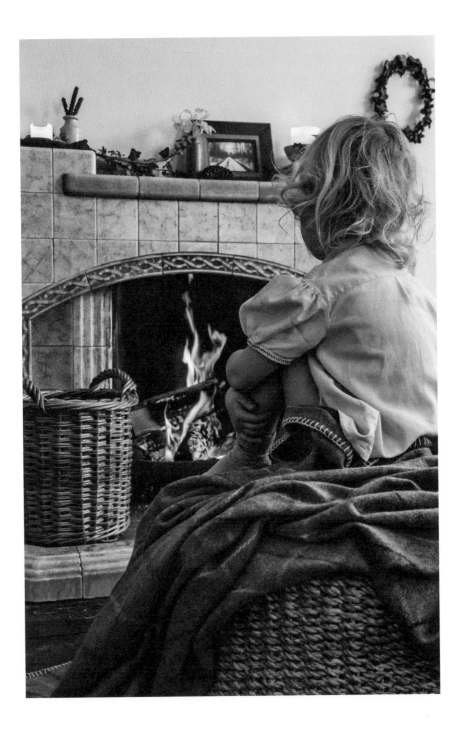

on household chores and hobbies, rather than the preferred pastimes of today, including browsing the internet and binge-watching TV shows.

While it is easy to look with nostalgia at days gone by, it is evident that there are lots of things we can learn about slow living and simplifying from previous generations. When I think about how my grandmother lived day-to-day, it is easy to see why she was good at appreciating the simple things and finding joy in life. My grandmother lived with her mum and seven siblings in a three-bedroom terrace house in Tooting, South London. She shared a bedroom with three sisters, and at her first job (at a department store on Oxford Street), she had to use the toilets in the nearest Tube station.

Without the basic luxuries we have today, people had gratitude for the things we take for granted. People were also more likely to be thoughtful with their choices, even small decisions, such as correspondence. It takes more time and effort to write a letter and post it, so naturally one would have put thought into any communication—it wasn't even easy to make a phone call.

By looking to the past and reflecting on how folks used to live, what lessons can we learn to guide us into the future? Wouldn't it be great if we could combine the wonderful things that make our lives easier in the twenty-first century with age-old traditions and ideas that better support our overall well-being?

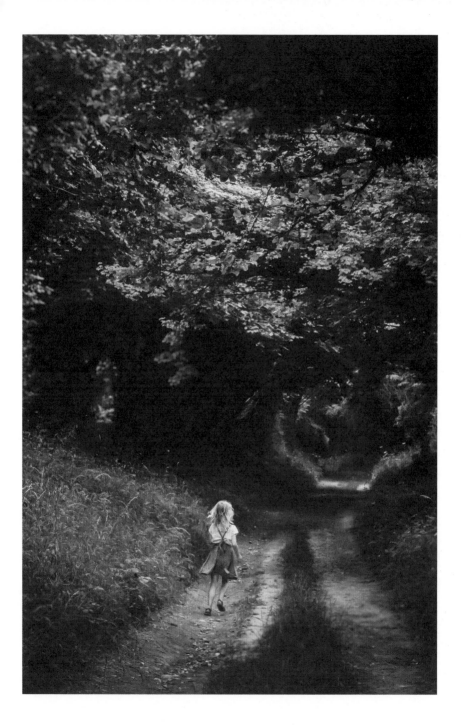

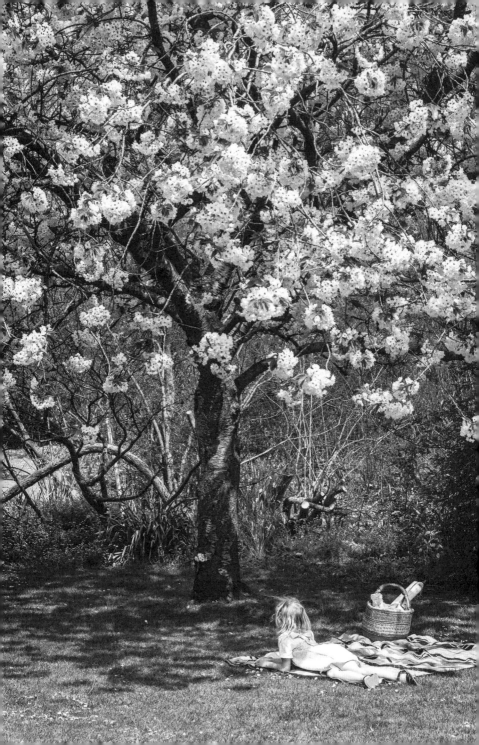

The Challenges of Our Modern Age

With the demands of twenty-first-century life, no wonder people are looking for alternative ways to live. For me, slow and simple living encompasses all the fundamental values that help my family live a more wholehearted life, from being connected to the present moment to appreciating the little things, and taking time to enjoy and celebrate life. Of course, there are many things that can hinder us on our quest to live more slowly, including the glorification of being "busy," consumer culture and materialism, and our digital age and virtual consumption, all things that we need to evaluate in our lives and decide whether we want and/or need a lifestyle change.

THE GLORIFICATION OF "BUSY"

Society seems to think success is directly correlated to how busy we are. When someone asks how one is doing, it is a standard twenty-first-century response to say "busy." We wear it like a badge of honor, taking pride in the fact that being busy implies that we are important.

This glorification of "busy" and the association of being "busy" with being "successful" is a dangerous equivalence, which inevitably has a negative effect on one's mental well-being. We can't be busy every hour of every day, so when do we stop? How will we know when we have reached the limit of our busyness and the peak of our success? If we aren't achieving anything, does that mean we're failing? The logic is unsustainable, and once we link feeling successful with being busy, finding contentment with our life becomes more of a challenge.

It is also amplified by social networks encouraging us to give status updates and let people know what we are "doing" all the time, as if "resting" isn't a valid pastime. People also only tend to share the positive stuff—their achievements and acquisitions. This leaves an area of life experiences that don't fit into that "picture-perfect" portrait of existence. Comparatively, it can leave us feeling like our lives don't quite measure up.

There is a deep fear that if we stopped being busy, for just a moment, we would be confronted by silence, and even more terrifying, we would have to face the fact that perhaps what we are "busy" doing isn't actually that important at all.

We need to remember that success doesn't just have to be defined by the big moments in our lives or by collecting material possessions. There can be great significance in the small, quiet moments and in life's little details. If we stop to think about it, there are other ways to evaluate how successful our lives are: the connections we make with others, how much love and happiness we inspire, the impact we have on our surroundings. By altering our definition of success, we will naturally slow down the pace of our days. By being realistic about what it means to be busy and by learning to relish the small, simple pleasures along the way, we can all find more meaning and joy in our lives.

CONSUMER CULTURE AND MATERIALISM

Consumer culture and buying material possessions are a fundamental part of society and how we live today. How we shop and consume things has changed dramatically over the last one hundred years, with shopping and buying material items becoming entangled with our identities and social statuses. We are used to consuming things at a rapid rate, not only in terms of our shopping habits and the products we buy, but also in how we consume information—pretty much anything is available at all hours of the day. If we want to live more slowly and simply, we must carefully examine and understand our consumer culture. In order to gain a greater understanding of why we consume things the way we do, it is really helpful to look back at why and how we have ended up with these current consumer habits.

The idea of buying things to achieve social status started in the 1920s, when Edward Bernays, the "father of public relations," came up with the concept of "aspirational marketing." Through his work with propaganda during the First World War, he understood how the minds of the masses could be manipulated through messages and advertising, and how powerful this was. It was during this time when society really began to "buy" into the product, along with the lifestyle attached to the product, and, most importantly, the idea that a product could make our lives better and more complete.

Soon after, the ideal of the American dream was born: regardless of social or financial status, anyone could work hard and climb the social ladder. Originally, the American dream was more about opportunity and less about material possessions; however, as consumerism developed, so did the American dream. What followed were marketing strategies designed to persuade people to consume more and more, from "planned obsolescence," where things (e.g., light bulbs and printer cartridges) are purposefully made to have a short life to encourage people to buy more (therefore, kickstarting the economy), to "perceived obsolescence," where the product (e.g., smartphones) still works, but it is no longer cool or relevant—it simply goes out of style. Whether or not an item is "in fashion" or "in style" remains the driving force behind consumerism.

One of the reasons that consumerism has become such a fundamental part of our society is the fact that shopping and buying things gives us a sense of identity, and most importantly, our sense of worth comes from the "stuff" we consume. Often this is fueled by the idea that something is lacking from within, and whatever we consume can fill that void and fix us. "The stuff props up our identity."[1] This is particularly apparent in the way women are

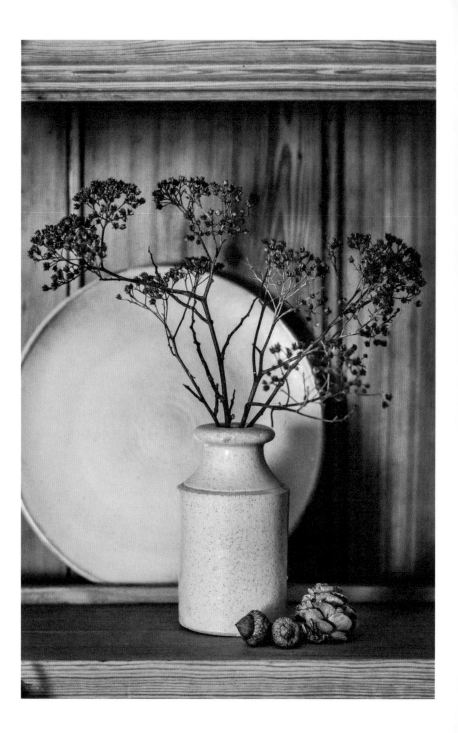

marketed to, as magazines are good at showing them impossibly perfect ideals, and with the turn of a page, showing them products that will help them attain this unrealistic definition of "beauty," whether it is clothing, beauty products, or home decor.

It is also a common misconception that material possessions are directly related to making us happy, with many of us even using shopping and consuming things to avoid difficult situations in our lives. It is easy to get caught in the loop of working to earn money, to buy material possessions (that fuel the economy), to improve social status and happiness. But, of course, material possessions and consuming things don't actually do this. Study after study shows us that experiences, not things, make us happy.[2]

Buying stuff can be fun, but it is important to notice what is motivating you to shop and consume—whether you are buying something because it is an essential item or whether it is a treat or luxury, providing a boost for your sense of identity and self-worth. It is also important to realize that even essential purchases are still wrapped up with our sense of self. Actually separating our consumer choices from our sense of identity is difficult, but having an awareness of the industry and how we are marketed to gives us the understanding to make more conscious choices.

That said, many of us are beginning to realize that the way we consume material possessions today simply is unsustainable for our planet. In order to initiate change, we must be aware of and take responsibility for our part in the consumer chain. By being thoughtful about our purchases, we will naturally begin to consider the environmental and the ethical impact that an item has on others and the planet. We must not underestimate the power we have as consumers to encourage change through the choices we make.

THE ART OF WAITING

There is an art to waiting for things, but it is becoming an unfamiliar concept to many of us in our consumer culture of instant gratification. We have become so used to having everything immediately accessible that we have forgotten how to patiently look forward to something and savor the suspense. By intentionally absorbing something at a slower pace, our enjoyment of it increases. Along with the buildup, excitement, and anticipation of the event, we are able to soak up as much joy as possible by being really present.

Our mood improves by having things to look forward to; these don't need to be big, extraordinary events but can be really simple pleasures, from our favorite TV show airing once a week (as opposed to binge-watching back-to-back episodes) to spending some time cooking and planning a simple lunch, then enjoying eating it with family and friends.

THE DIGITAL AGE AND
VIRTUAL CONSUMPTION

Consumption is not only limited to shopping for and buying material possessions. With everything accessible at a swipe of the finger, it is harder than ever before to live in the present moment. We all have a little distraction in our pocket that is constantly competing for our attention. Previously, when we would have been doing nothing, we now have the option to do a whole menu of things: text, check our email, catch up on social media, or browse the bottomless resource that is the internet. With so many choices in front of us, it can leave us feeling like there isn't any free time to simply switch off and not do anything. It is fundamental to be able to sit in silence with ourselves, but with temptation literally at hand, many of us have turned to reaching for our phones as a distraction.

Of course, the digital age has brought wonderful advances that we should celebrate. We now have much more flexibility and diversity in how we work, communicate, and connect with others; however, living slowly becomes more of a challenge because of this digital age that we live in. Virtual consumption and the wealth of information that is readily available to us at any time of the day means that moments of stillness have become few and far between.

It is really easy to waste a lot of time on our phones and not really get anything done, which results in us spending more time on our phones than we would ideally like to. One of the main reasons we check our phones a lot is due to notifications. Notifications make us feel good; we get gratification from the sense of connection that a text message or a Facebook or Instagram "like" provides. Our phones buzzing all the time from our various notifications reinforces our self-worth. It makes us feel like people care about what we have to say, and in turn that people care about us. Additionally, when we receive a notification, we get a little dopamine hit.

Dopamine is a chemical responsible for transmitting signals between brain cells. It is required for lots of complex brain functions, including motivation, attention, mood, and, in this instance, rewarding experiences. There is a lot of information about how a spike in dopamine can create pleasure or motivation, but actually it is something called "opioids" that gives us that giddy feeling. More accurately, dopamine is responsible for the anticipation of a reward that our brain has associated with a certain activity, and most importantly, it then has our brain seeking out that specific activity over and over again. For example, when posting a picture to Instagram, we have learned that we will get a reward—a dopamine hit—when we check our notifications. It is easy to see why we can become addicted to checking our phones. If one notification can give us a little spike in dopamine and the pleasure-filled chemicals, opioids, imagine what hundreds of "likes" on one photo can do.

Behavior is, of course, very complex, and there are many factors that affect the decisions we make. To blame checking social networks every five minutes on dopamine would be a huge oversimplification. It is also important to acknowledge that a lot of online activities, especially where social networks are concerned, are designed to keep us engaged and using their platforms for as long as possible. These big companies make money from us using their sites, and they employ people whose jobs are to figure out how to keep us engaged and spending more time on their specific network or platform.

Understanding the context of why we constantly (and even unknowingly) reach for our phones and why we check our notifications can be the first step toward changing our online behavior and habits. As we move further into this century, technology is only going to continue to develop and the amount of information that is available to increase. It is, therefore, important that we put some clear boundaries in place and are thoughtful about how we use our phones, tablets, and computers. By being intentional with how we use our time and how and when we access the wealth of information that is available to us, we can strike a healthy balance between taking advantage of the flexibility of this wonderful technology while also making sure we don't allow it to overtake our moments of stillness.

Digital Detox

Here are some simple boundaries you can put in place to help you create some distance between you and your phone to make more space for those slow and wholehearted moments.

Designate a phone zone.
When you are at home, designate a spot to leave your phone so that it is not constantly "on you." Ideally, place it somewhere that you have to get up and walk to in order to pick up your phone. By consciously having to go to the area to check your phone, you will become aware of how often you have the urge to look.

Set intentional online time.
Have designated times when you are "online" and when you are "offline." I enjoy engaging with my community on Instagram and have specific times, mostly evenings, where I spend focused time posting and commenting. Then the next evening, I will take a break and won't open the app at all. Remember that on the evenings you are not online, you can leave your phone in another room (or in your designated spot); otherwise, temptation can become too great to just have a quick check.

Turn off notifications.
Turn off push notifications and only check your social networks and email at designated times—this way, you will not be constantly distracted or pulled into the online world.

Time yourself. If you find that you lose all sense of time when on social networks, try setting a timer on your phone for fifteen minutes, then make sure you switch off when the fifteen minutes are up.

Respect your sacred sleep.
Try making your bedroom a phone-free zone, leaving your phone outside the bedroom overnight. We go to bed to rest and sleep, and that time to rejuvenate is essential for our health and well-being. Again, if your phone isn't within reaching distance, it removes the temptation to just have a last-minute look before bed or first thing when you wake up.

Implement gentle transitions. Try not looking at your phone for the first hour of each day and for at least an hour before bedtime. We can't expect our bodies and minds to process anything until we are properly awake, so give yourself a gentle start and a chance to fully wake up. Equally, at the end of the day, a gentle wind-down is helpful. It is important to prepare your body and mind for sleep, and looking at your phone just before bed will only stimulate your mind.

Detox weekly. Once a week, make sure you avoid social networks and being online for at least twenty-four hours. Several times a year, try a total detox for longer periods. This time offline (even just twenty-four hours) makes such a big difference to our mental well-being. It gives our minds time to reset and allows us to lift our gaze and focus on other things.

Make it positive. If you are finding that when you are on social networks, it isn't making you feel good about yourself, then take a step back. Social networks should be a way for us to feel connected and inspired, and if they are not doing at least one of those things, then it is time to question why we are logging on.

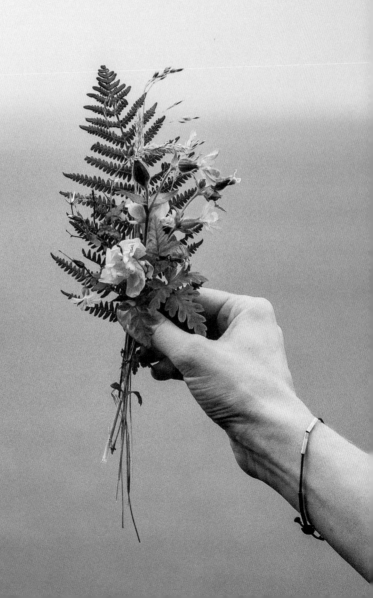

Time

....

We would all like more time to do as we please, including time to slow down, relax, enjoy life, and connect with the ones we love. Time can seem so elusive; it can both drag and fly by. Time is a resource that we simply cannot get back. Once it has gone, it is gone. No wonder a lot of us are obsessed with being as productive as possible with our time. Perhaps we feel that there aren't enough hours in the day to complete all the things that need doing. Maybe that's why we clock-watch and cram every minute of the day with tasks. If we are not achieving things and crossing them off our to-do lists, many of us feel like we have wasted our day.

VALUING OUR TIME

We've all heard the saying "time is money"; however, if we valued our time in terms of a monetary amount per hour, we would miss out on many of life's simple joys. There are lots of things we do with our time that are extremely valuable and worthwhile but won't earn us any money: sleeping, reading a bedtime story to your children, sharing a meal with friends and family. Money isn't the real value of time and it can be dangerous to begin to think of our time in that way.

It can be helpful to think about our time from a more philosophical view: How can we use our time in a way that makes our lives meaningful? What are we here for? What is our purpose? What is important to us? What are our priorities?

We must also be aware that the choices we make about how we use and manage our time has a ripple effect on those around us. It doesn't just impact our lifestyles and well-being, but it also impacts our families, our communities, and the planet. For example, we can have a negative effect on the planet if we feel we are too busy to recycle, or if we tell ourselves we don't have time to stop and play with our children, or we don't have time to volunteer or help with any school or community projects.

We must make sure we acknowledge how precious our time is to us, as it will undoubtedly affect what we choose to do with that time. If we want others to value our time, we must lead by example and commit to valuing our personal time too. Many of us don't set clear boundaries with our time: we say "yes" to every-thing, are always available, and often value others' time above our own.

Finally, we must not underestimate how being inten-tional with our time is instrumental in slowing down. If we can learn to focus on one specific task in a mindful way, we are going to be able to fully absorb ourselves in what we are doing and make the most of our time.

MANAGING OUR TIME

Because of this desire to maximize our time and there-fore our productivity, "time management" has become a popular topic. There are numerous books, articles, blogs, and podcasts on time management and produc-tivity techniques that are full of suggestions on how to get the most out of our time, from time-boxing tasks and making "do-not-do lists" to avoiding procrastina-tion and practicing motivational thinking. In fact, it is easy to get lost in a sea of time-management self-help articles and feel overwhelmed by which techniques to

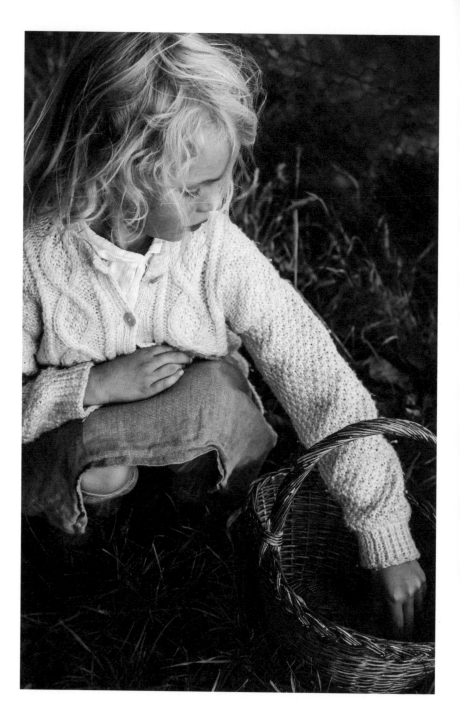

try. Writing a simple to-do list has even become a complex art form, with rules and advice on how to write the best list to increase your productivity.

Of course, it makes sense to spend some time putting good systems in place that work for you, as in the long run, they will save you time, help you be more efficient, and reduce your stress levels. What can be helpful is to think of time management along the lines of working smarter. Start by simplifying what you do and prioritizing what's important. Here are a few key things to look out for when thinking about how to manage your time.

Focusing on what is urgent as opposed to what is important, and focusing on the trivial instead of the meaningful. One of the most famous time-management tools is the Eisenhower principle, which was developed by the US president Dwight D. Eisenhower. He famously said, "I have two kinds of problems, the urgent and the important. The urgent are not important, and the important are never urgent." Things that feel urgent make us prioritize them, whether the task is actually urgent or not. This perceived urgency makes us want to complete the task quickly, even if the task is trivial. The physical bodily reaction we have to the urgency can be all-consuming and hard to ignore. It is almost impossible to argue with such an automatic primal response, even though our minds know that the task is, in fact, inconsequential.

Hurrying has become a default setting for many because we feel that we have too much to do. If we have a lot to do in a short amount of time, the obvious response it to try to do everything more quickly. However, hurrying is the poison of productivity, and the big flaw of having a hurried mental approach is that it creates a scarcity mind-set that there are not enough hours in the day. Approaching our tasks and workday feeling that there is insufficient time increases our stress levels. Hurrying can turn into putting pressure on ourselves to get stuff done, which then grows into stress and anxiety that festers and expands until we are overwhelmed.

Multitasking hinders us from being intentional with our time, resulting in inefficiency and poorer end results. When people are really busy, it is easy to see why they fall into the trap of multitasking. Our brains have evolved to just focus on one thing at a time, and it is only the demands of twenty-first-century life that have us convinced we can multitask.[3] Encouraging this behavior is a cognitive illusion that we are doing a great job even when we are not. In his book *The Organized Mind: Thinking Straight in the Age of Information Overload*, Daniel Levitin explains that our attention is easily hijacked by the novelty of a shiny new distraction/task/stimuli, like checking Facebook or answering an email: "Multitasking creates a dopamine-addiction feedback loop, effectively rewarding the brain for losing focus and for constantly searching for external stimulation."[4] The reality is, though, that we use more energy switching from one task to another. Every time we cognitively change gears to focus our attention on something else, we use up oxygenated glucose. Levitin expounds, "And the kind of rapid, continual shifting we do with multitasking causes the brain to burn through fuel so quickly that we feel exhausted and disoriented even after a short time. We've literally depleted the nutrients in our brain."[5] In fact, multitasking means we become overloaded with information. Making decisions is also hard on our neural resources—even little decisions, like "Should I reply to this email?" The more we switch from task to task, the more decisions we are faced with.

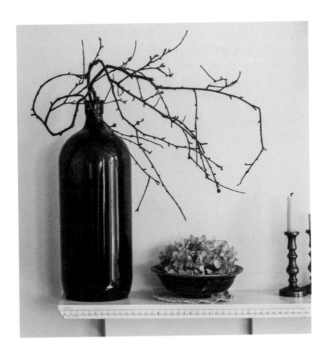

Working Smarter

Here are some time-management ideas that will help you work smarter. By spending some time thinking about how you approach your day and tasks, you will be able to work more efficiently and reduce your stress levels.

Focus on what is important, not what feels urgent. Even though the urgent items feel pressing, it is more valuable for you to complete the important tasks.

Resist the trap of multitasking. A more efficient use of our energy and time is to focus on just one individual thing (monotasking). By doing so, you will be more productive, as well as less tired and neurochemically depleted at the end of the task.

Avoid hurrying and be intentional with your time. Hurrying is the poison to productivity, creates a scarcity mind-set, and increases stress levels. By dedicating some time and energy to thinking about how to approach your day and schedule, you will alleviate that sense of hurrying and allow yourself to sink into each part of your day with enjoyment. Plus, you are much more likely to create a conducive atmosphere for productivity and creativity.

Define your purpose and priorities. By having a clear understanding of your purpose and priorities, you can make sure that you do the important work first when you have the most energy. Save the small tasks that aren't so important for the end of the day.

Time-box tasks. Give each task on your to-do list a guesstimation of how long the task will take. You can also section your tasks into small, medium, and large based on how much time they will take. Doing this will help you use your time more efficiently.

Batch similar tasks. This can be as simple as answering your emails in one sitting and having a couple hours to work on your accounts to separating tasks according to whether they have a similar focus and attentional set. Some tasks require you to think about the big picture, some require you to be detailed oriented, and others require you to simply focus on getting the bulk of the work done. By working from the same attentional set, where your level of focus is consistent, you will get more done and finish with more energy.

Understand the difference between tasks, projects, and goals. A task is a small, identifiable piece of work; a project is a series of tasks that result in a specific target; and a goal is a "big-picture" ambition or objective.

Add only small, manageable, and specific things to your to-do list. If you add something that is too big, like "write a book," of course, it is never going to get done. A more appropriate task would be "write outline for book," or "write five hundred words for chapter one."

OUR PURPOSE AND PRIORITIES

For many of us, much of our week is scheduled with school functions, work, and various commitments, leaving little free time. The fact that our days can be so heavily scheduled means the week moves at a quick pace, and there is little opportunity to be spontaneous or follow our heart's desire. When trying to slow down the week's pace, I have found it necessary to make sure to block out time where nothing is scheduled. As a family, I have found that we need at least one whole day with no time restraints at all. It is a great way to take the pressure off, reconnect with and indulge that inner voice, and do exactly what we feel like.

When thinking about our time and schedules, we need to acknowledge that we cannot do it all. It is important to be mindful about what and how many activities we choose to include in our weekly routines. Two words that I frequently revisit in my slow-living journey are purpose and priorities. Our **purpose** is what is motivating and driving us to make the choices we make. It is important to understand our purpose when looking at the bigger picture of our lives and the plans and goals we have, as well as understanding what our purpose is for the day-to-day tasks. Figuring out our **priorities** really helps us work out what we do (and do not) have time for. Again, this works on the larger scale of looking at our life priorities, as well as the smaller tasks on our to-do lists. By working out what things are the most important, we can decide which tasks and activities we are happy to let go of. I have found that using "joy" as a guide is a really helpful way to hone in on which activities are important to us and our families. If it isn't bringing joy into our lives, then why is it an additional part of our weekly routine?

By spending some time thinking about our purpose, we will begin to uncover what is motivating us to move at a slower speed. By choosing our priorities, we will learn to leave the trivial stuff behind and begin to focus on the meaningful things in our lives.

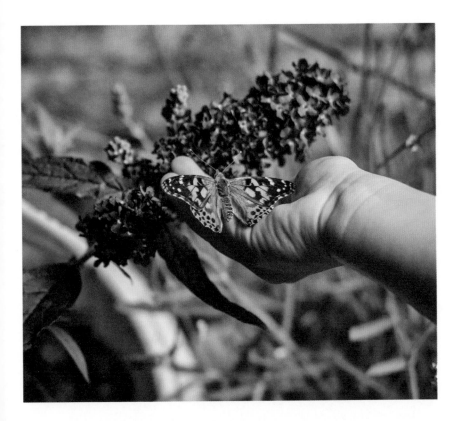

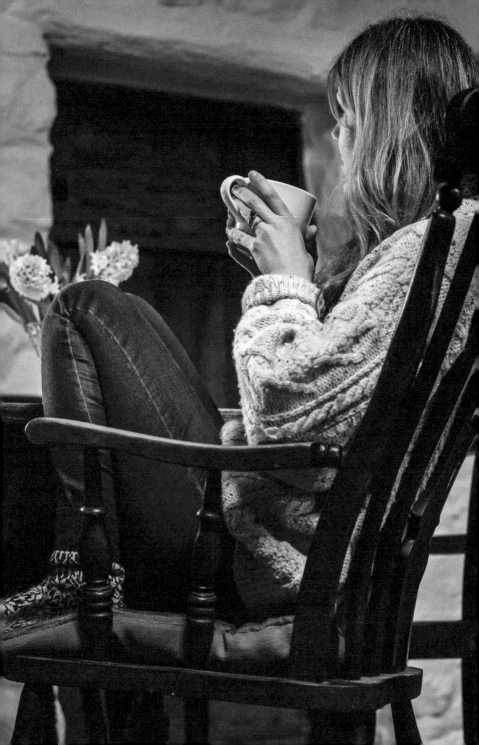

Learning to Nurture Ourselves

···········

Learning to nurture and really look after ourselves is one of life's essential lessons, yet many of us find it difficult to do. However, in recent years, "self-care" has become an increasingly popular topic and a growing industry. We are also beginning to understand how far the term "well-being" stretches and what it encompasses, realizing that it is linked to our personal happiness, as well as a healthy body, mind, and spirit. It is crucial to carve out time in our week to tend to ourselves; otherwise, we are left running on empty. If we do not make time to look after our well-being, then we cannot be present for those around us, fulfill our responsibilities, and live a wholehearted life.

MAKING TIME FOR OURSELVES

In order to nurture our bodies, minds, and general well-being, it is important to prioritize time for ourselves and our self-care. Often, we put ourselves at the bottom of the list, though we inherently know we need time to take care of ourselves. Yet, we can feel guilty about taking this "me time." How do we justify an hour taking a bath when there is a big list of tasks that "need" to get done?

Often, these ideals are heavily linked to our self-esteem, self-worth, and especially our self-compassion. These thought patterns and beliefs have been established over years, if not decades, so adjusting our thinking—and altering our habits—will take some time. The first step is to acknowledge that as adults, our bodies and minds still need support and nourishment to thrive and develop. Here are a few ways to make time for yourself.

Redefine which weekly tasks are essential. There will undoubtedly be things on your to-do list that at first glance seem to be important, but when you take a moment to reevaluate, you can recognize that, comparatively, they are not as important as your well-being.

Assess the toll of emotional labor. It is important not to underestimate how much time and energy is taken up from thinking about things that need to get done or that are scheduled, like who has what activity after school, what the family is having for dinner, whose birthday it is this month, and whether the toilet-paper roll needs replacing. A lot of this "work" often goes unnoticed. By acknowledging how much time this takes up, you can look at ways to enlist assistance and support from your family to help share the load.

Identify and acknowledge "slow moments." Think about what you do in your week that makes you breathe out and go a little slower—simple things like listening to music, making a cup of tea, gardening, or going for a walk. Whatever they are, make sure you identify and acknowledge what those tasks and activities are and then sprinkle them throughout your week. These are your "slow moments," and they will become an essential part of your slow-living process.

Slow Moments

Slow moments are anything you do that help you to slow down and feel calm. There are most likely certain activities you do on a daily basis that you automatically find comforting—things that make you breathe a little deeper and help your mind relax. Here are some examples of slow moments:

taking a bath

going for a walk

listening to music

puttering around your home

gardening

knitting

reading a book

playing (see page 56)

baking

Try to go through the next few days and impartially observe what you do in a day. Where do you find these slow moments and how? Are there days when you don't experience any slow moments?

EMBRACING SELF-COMPASSION

When learning to nurture ourselves, a pivotal quality is self-compassion. In its purest form, "self-compassion" is about loving and relating to ourselves kindly. Most of us are good at having compassion for others, but having compassion for ourselves is just as important. Self-esteem has been the favored pop psychology topic of the last few decades, and Western culture understands the importance of supporting our self-esteem; however, we are still learning to recognize the importance of self-compassion. Dr. Kristine Neff, one of the leading researchers of self-compassion, points out some interesting distinctions between self-esteem and self-compassion, with the main difference being that self-esteem is contingent on certain things like being exceptional at something, or comparatively better than others, whereas self-compassion is steadfast regardless of whether you succeed or fail.

Self-compassion is not generally encouraged in Western culture, and many of us have misconceptions about how being more compassionate toward ourselves could have a negative impact on our attitude and behaviors. It is common to think that self-compassion makes us weak, and that we need to be tough to cope with life; in actuality, practicing self-compassion develops our inner strength and resilience. Another common misconception is that being hard on ourselves is what drives us to succeed; however, self-criticism is not an effective motivator. Many think that if we are compassionate toward ourselves, we are actually indulging in self-pity and that it will lead to laziness; instead, practicing self-compassion encourages us to think about our long-term health and well-being, and we learn to acknowledge that life is hard for everyone. Finally, we may feel that it is selfish to think about ourselves in a compassionate way; however, giving to ourselves allows us to be able to give to others.

Dr. Neff says that there are three pillars of self-compassion: self-kindness, common humanity, and mindfulness.[6] The first pillar is simply talking and relating to ourselves kindly and learning to not judge ourselves. For the second pillar, we need to understand that we are not alone in any suffering, and that imperfection is part of the shared human experience. And regarding the third pillar, when we are suffering, we need to acknowledge that, and then mindfully observe our response with perspective. It is important not to overidentify or suppress our emotions in order to begin to process what we are feeling. Dr. Neff explains, "Individuals who are more self-compassionate tend to have great happiness, life satisfaction, and motivation, better relationships and physical health d less anxiety and depression."[7]

Start by ask g yourself, "What do I need?" If we can begin to treat ourselves like a dear friend, and learn to talk to ourselves kindly, then we can lay a stable foundation for a healthy relationship with ourselves.

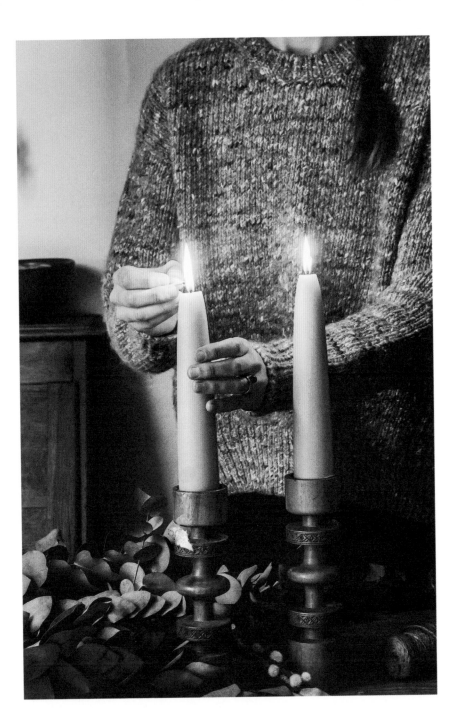

PLAY

Of course, rest and relaxation help us slow down, but another key component to slowing down is play. It is just one of the many examples of things we can re-learn from our children. It's second nature for children to play; they instinctively know how to throw themselves into games and use their imaginations. However, as adults, we often have forgotten how to lose ourselves in play.

It is undeniable how much children learn through play and using their imaginations; they develop their language skills, social and emotional skills, thinking skills, physical skills, self-confidence, and self-esteem. For adults, play can relieve stress, stimulate the mind and boost creativity, help with problem-solving, and improve their connections and relationships with others.

What constitutes as play can be hard to define, and, of course, what feels like play differs from person to person. Play is most definitely a process, and although multifarious, these activities have a few qualities in common: a sense of freedom to experiment and try out things without the merit of success or failure, space to get lost in the activity with no clock-watching, and no expectation of a productive outcome or result (though it might result in something productive). According to Dr. Stuart Brown, the founder of The National Institute for Play, "If its purpose is more important than the act of doing it, it's probably not play."[8]

There are many ways for adults to access that sense of play, whether it is object play, social play, rough-and-tumble play, spectator play, or imaginative solo play. Creative play can be a particularly wonderful way for adults to have a chance to explore and experiment, and to tap into that sense of freedom. It's very satisfying to get lost in the flow of a task where you are solely absorbed in the activity you are doing. This flow also helps you stay in the present moment of each part of the task. These days, there are not many things we do where our minds are purely focused on one individual thing without lots of distractions.

The great thing about making something or being physically active is that by letting our hands and bodies move, we can slow down our minds. Play allows us to lose ourselves, along with our sense of time, which is beneficial to our psychological well-being. It is a mistake to think of play as some sort of rehearsal for adult activity, or to just confine play to that of a hobby. Play is nourishing, and the research of Dr. Brown, who is a leading expert on the science of play and how important it is for our happiness and well-being, teaches us that play has a significant biological place in our lives (just as sleep and dreams do).

DAYDREAMING AND BOREDOM

We also need to allow ourselves space to daydream for our mental well-being. It is vital to have time when we are not thinking about anything productive but just letting our thoughts seamlessly float through a stream of consciousness. We all need moments in our day when our minds are relaxed and disengaged from things. Daniel Levitin, an award-winning neuroscientist and author, explains, "Daydreaming mode . . . turns out to be restorative. It's like hitting the reset button in your brain."[9]

If you can remember life before mobile phones existed, you will know what it is like to sit on a train and have nothing to do but gaze out the window or read a book. You will also have experienced standing in a queue for something and getting lost in your own thoughts and daydreams. Because of the wonderful advances with technology, potentially there is a whole generation that will not have those experiences to draw from unless we encourage them to unplug and indulge in a bit of good old-fashioned daydreaming.

Time seems different when you are daydreaming—slower somehow—and how we use our minds while daydreaming is very different from how we use them during dedicated focus. When we daydream, we are playful, intuitive, and relaxed.[10] Perhaps that is why creative and inspirational ideas are often born from daydreaming. We need to allow our minds space to ruminate and for our imaginations to be free. Only then can the gap be filled with a creative idea or answer. According to Daniel Levitin, "Creative solutions often arise from allowing a sequence of altercations between dedicated focus and daydreaming."[11]

In fact, I would take it one step further and say that not only do we need to daydream more, but we also need to allow ourselves and our children to get bored. Just like with daydreaming, boredom encourages our minds to wander, and the natural lull allows our energy to replenish. It also encourages creative thinking. Remember when you were a child and you would say you were bored? What followed would be an interval where you had to use your initiative and imagination to think of something creative to occupy yourself with.

It is evident that time spent daydreaming or being bored is essential for our mental well-being, and that now more than ever, when there are many distractions to keep our brains occupied and engaged, we have to be more mindful and intentional about making sure we have gaps in our days to let our minds slow down.

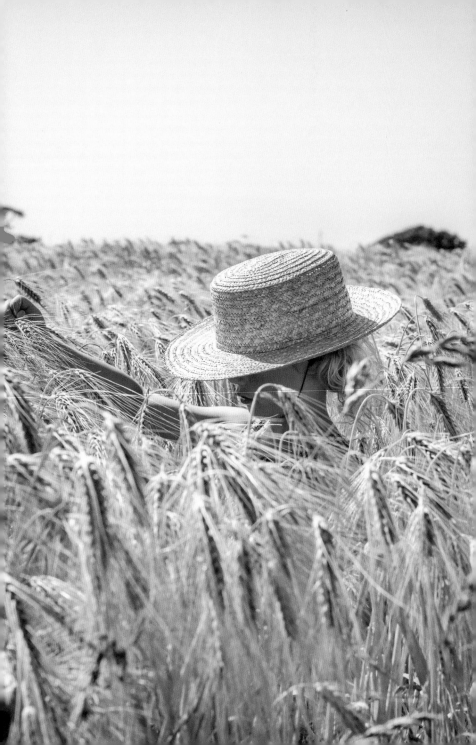

Well-Being

BODY

....

We often do all our "thinking" with our minds, even though our bodies possess inherent intelligence. They often know what is best for us: when we need to rest, when we need fresh air and exercise. If we take just a moment to think about all the amazing things our bodies do—all the movements, automated bodily functions, brain processing, tissue growth and repairs, hormone releases, etc.—then it makes sense for us to put some time aside to take care of and look after them. By slowing down things, we are able to listen to our bodies with more clarity and develop our body-mind connection, which in turn allows us to feel connected to our "self" in new ways.

LEARNING TO LISTEN TO OUR BODIES

For many, the desire to slow down comes from listening to a faint call from deep within the body. We instinctively know that something is not right—that the pace of life is too fast. Ignoring or silencing this voice, because we are too busy, is only a temporary fix. That raw impulse to slow down will not disappear; instead, if we can learn how to tune in to our bodies and converse with this voice, we can allow it to guide us.

Learning to listen to our bodies is a fundamental life skill, but what exactly do we mean by "listening"? We receive messages from our bodies all the time. Physical messages, such as hunger, thirst, and pain, are often the first signals we are aware of. Our body also sends us subtle messages, signals in the form of emotions and feelings. Listening encourages us to become more aware of the general sensations in our bodies. Importantly, it helps us identify what tension feels like, and in contrast, what relaxation feels like. It also helps us distinguish between good pain versus bad pain and tune in to our emotional intelligence, which improves our intuition. However, it is easy to miss these subtle messages when we have so many distractions in our lives that hinder us from listening to our bodies. These distractions range from clutter in our home and overscheduled weeks to information overload and virtual consumption.

When we are aware of what our bodies are feeling, many of us have become good at suppressing these messages and feelings. It is understandable why we numb ourselves; some of the feelings that come our way, like sadness, grief, and loneliness, aren't much fun to experience. However, there are several problems that come from quashing how we really feel. Firstly, we cannot pick and choose which emotions we want to feel. A numbing of one, leads to a numbing of everything. If we suppress sadness, we also never get to experience the brilliance of joy, or the intense pleasure of passion. Secondly, once we start to shut down the conversations and the ability to understand the messages our bodies send us, we struggle to really know what we want and need. By learning to nurture ourselves and by being more self-compassionate we will begin to change the way we interact with ourselves. With time, we can gradually learn to open up a dialogue with our body, develop self-trust, and allow ourselves to experience the whole gamut of our emotions.

The Benefits of Listening to Your Body

Here are some of the benefits of learning to listen to your body and developing your body-mind connection.

Better health. Overall, you will feel better, as you will have an increased awareness of your body and will recognize when you need to rest and do less.

Increased intuition. By listening to your body, you can increase your intuition and become more insightful, which in turn helps you understand what you really want (your heart's desire).

Less aches. Once you are able to converse with your body and understand where any aches are coming from, you will also know what you can do to help improve them, such as posture adjustments or stretches and exercises.

Discernment of good pain versus bad pain. If you have ever heard the phrase "good pain" and not understood what it meant, you will start to be able to notice the difference between different types of pain. For example, when doing physical activity or stretching, you will be aware of pain that is expected and productive and of pain that has a detrimental effect and means you are damaging something. It is helpful to be able to distinguish between these two different types of pain.

Better understanding of stress and anxiety. By becoming curious about how your body and mind work, you will gain a deeper understanding of why and how you become stressed and anxious, which in turn will help you know what you can do to alleviate such feelings.

Healthy relationship with food.
For many of us, our relationship with food can be complicated. Understanding when you are actually hungry and truly full is vital, along with deciphering what your body is craving and why, and then working out what your body actually needs.

Improved emotional intelligence. Emotions are complicated because they can feel so big and all-consuming when they are happening. Or alternatively, we are fearful of feeling too much, so we try to completely quash our emotions. It is important to acknowledge your emotions and understand that they will not magically disappear. It is also equally important to understand that your emotional response to something does not define who you are. You will start to observe your emotions and recognize them for what they are—just a response to something that will eventually fade. Once we understand that how we emotionally react to something isn't who we are and doesn't represent the truth, it will help us not to overidentify with our emotions.

Healthy relationships and boundaries. Becoming aware of taking on too much and people-pleasing will help you establish healthy boundaries. It is important to know when to say "no" in order to preserve your relationships.

More pleasure. Once you stop suppressing your feelings, you allow yourself to be open to the full spectrum of emotions, and therefore, will start to experience more pleasure and joy.

Self-trust. Once you start to believe and trust in the messages that come from your body and see the positive impact of listening to your body, you will gain more trust in yourself and the process. This in turn will help to alleviate general anxiety and self-doubt.

Increased autonomy. Once your self-trust grows, you will realize that you have the necessary tools within yourself to cope with life's challenges and are therefore able to navigate whatever comes your way.

THE BODY-MIND CONNECTION

By learning to listen to our bodies, we cannot help but explore the body-mind connection. The body-mind connection acknowledges that our minds have the ability to affect our bodies—our thoughts, feelings, and emotions can positively and negatively impact the way our bodies function. In reverse, our bodies also can affect our minds—what we eat and how much sleep we get affects our thoughts and how we feel.

This body-mind connection also helps us better understand how all the parts of our bodies fit together and move. Watching children move and play is so inspirational, as they instinctively know how to be connected to their bodies. As we age, our bodies become well worn and marked with our life experiences. We often learn bad habits in terms of movement and posture, and often become disconnected from our physical being. Spending time reconnecting the body and mind allows us to correct bad posture habits and helps us move more freely and with ease.

By slowing down and creating space to understand the body-mind connection and by listening to our bodies, we can live fuller lives. Paying attention to the messages our bodies send us positively impacts our well-being, from better health and less aches and pains to having a clearer understanding of stress and anxiety. If we allow them, our bodies can be great at guiding us to a more balanced way of life.

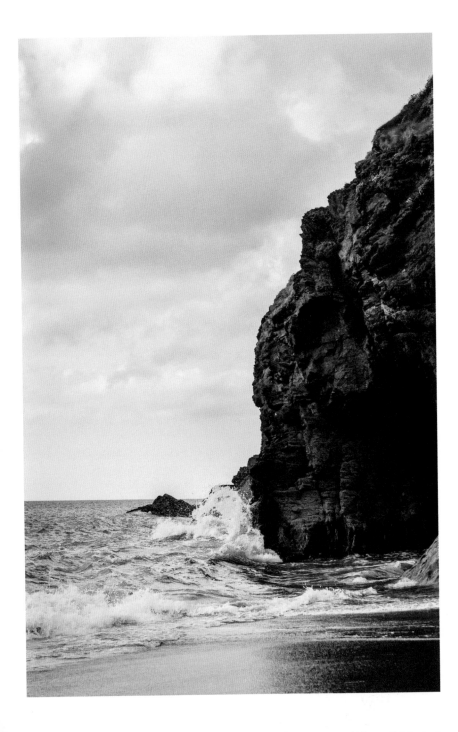

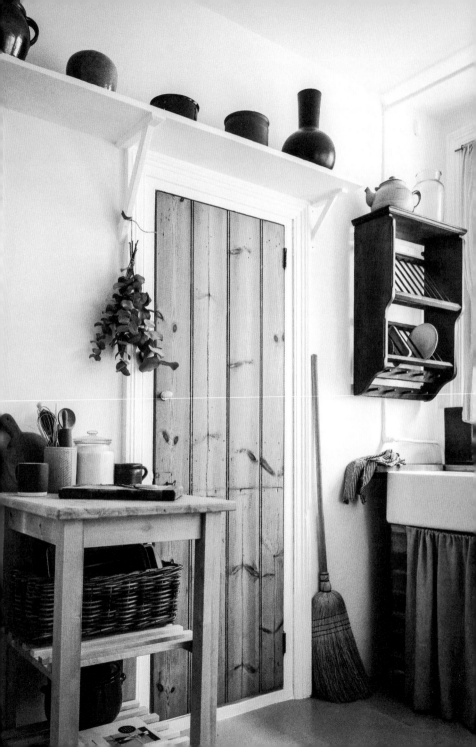

A Slow Home

....

Our homes and what we surround ourselves with are deeply intertwined with our slow-living experience. And it is essential to invest some time looking closely at our homes and whether we have them set up in a way that supports us and encourages a slower pace. How our homes feel, and the space around us, can make an impact on our well-being. A slow home can help us to connect deeply to ourselves and allow us to focus on the important things.

CREATING A SLOW HOME

When talking about creating a slow home, a good place to start is with simplifying our homes. Ideally, we want an environment that is easy to manage, comfortable, organized, and functional. There are three main areas you should focus on to achieve this: the design and decor of the space; the belongings that are in your home; and the habits, routines, and rhythms of the people who live within your home.

When looking at the **design and decor** of a home, it is crucial to think about how calm a room feels. The materials, colors, and fabrics that are used within the room, as well as the furniture and items, all feed into this. With the design of a slow home, there should be pockets of space to allow life to happen. Is there room for children to be creative and play? Is there a space that encourages rest? Finally, consider how ethical and natural your home is: Is it a space that nourishes your health and well-being?

Try to be thoughtful about the **belongings** within your home. It is helpful to adopt a conscious shopping habit and take time to think about whether you really "need" an item. A slow home takes time to come together, especially when purchasing key pieces like furniture—it is good to develop the patience to wait for the right piece of furniture to come along. It is also necessary to consider how well your belongings are organized. If things are a mess and jumbled up, it makes day-to-day living harder than necessary because you don't know where to find anything, and even more importantly, you don't know where to tidy things away. Of course, the fewer belongings you have in the first place, the less "stuff" there is to sort through.

Finally, to truly have a slow and simple home, we need to look beyond the decor and the things we own and focus on our **habits, routines, and rhythms**. By spending some time thinking about these things in regard to your home, you will be able to truly assess how slow your home is. Is there space for any calm pauses within your day? Think about how you can alter your routine to make space for some slow moments. Are there any negative habits surrounding how you live in your home that you can specifically look at to help your day flow more smoothly? For example, do you find yourself always in a rush in the morning? If so, perhaps you could improve your sleep routine at the end of the day so you go to bed earlier and more relaxed.

Of course, our daily rhythms are affected by our living space, and vice versa, but if we solely focus on our environment, we are only doing half the work. To make long-lasting, deep changes, we must look below the surface and tackle our routines, rhythms, and habits. Only then will we really be able to experience a slow and simple home.

SIMPLIFYING OUR BELONGINGS

It is important to be able to look around our homes and feel calm. If we are surrounded by clutter and mess all the time, it is bound to negatively impact our mood and well-being. By simplifying and getting rid of some of our belongings, life can feel lighter and easier to manage. Clearing the clutter helps improve day-to-day life because everything is organized and has its place. It also helps us to live in the present moment, free from distractions and any associated stress or guilt over the piles of "stuff."

When looking at simplifying what we own, sorting and organizing our things can feel like a massive task. For motivation, when clearing the clutter, it is good to have a specific intention to come back to, to help keep you focused on what you are doing and why. One approach is to have the intention to **get rid of needless things**; however, what we "need" can be subjective. We could arguably live without lots of the items we have in our homes, but by owning them, life seems more comfortable. Or we could set the intention to surround ourselves with things that **add value and joy**. Thinking about how much value a possession adds to your life can be really helpful when deciding what to let go of. For example,

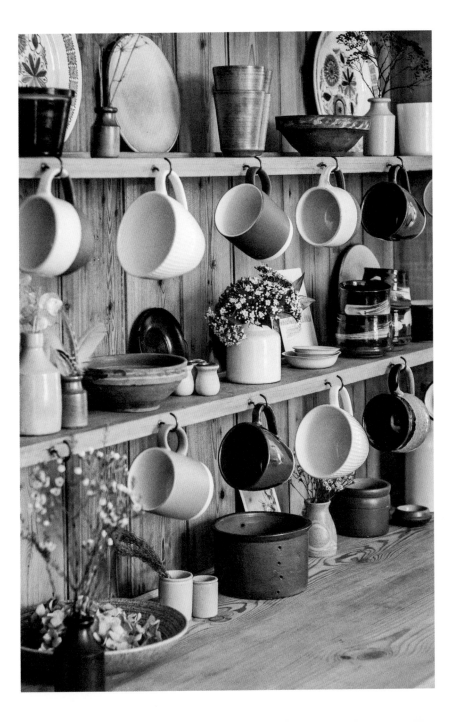

someone might own a collection of thousands of books, a piece of art, or a family heirloom that they don't really "need," but surely, such a treasured collection or item brings great value and joy into their lives—we all "need" a bit of that too. Whatever your intention, hold onto it when simplifying your belongings.

When sorting through items, it can be helpful to sort by category—clothes, books, paperwork. By piling all our items of a specific category in one space, we will realize how much "stuff" we actually have, which is another great way to motivate us to get rid of the excess. In fact, just the process of sorting through our belongings in this way provides a great opportunity to reevaluate things altogether. It helps us become aware of how much we consume and what items are really necessary.

Once we have sorted through all our belongings and have decided what we are happy to let go of, we must remember to rehome and recycle what we can. We want to try to avoid everything just ending up in landfill. Can any items be repurposed or donated to charity, and finally, can they be recycled?

It is also sensible to spend some time looking at how we store our possessions in the most effective way. It's comforting to know that every item has a specific home and a place to be put away. It makes it easier to keep the home tidy, which in turn means we are less stressed and more able to relax.

It can be easy to fall into the trap of constantly searching for more and more things, and the act of simplifying our belongings helps us appreciate what we have. Instead of being distracted by the clutter, we can better appreciate all the treasured and personal items we own. An uncluttered environment also allows us to tune in to the important stuff in life. We can focus on creating memories, being present, and enjoying all those wholehearted moments.

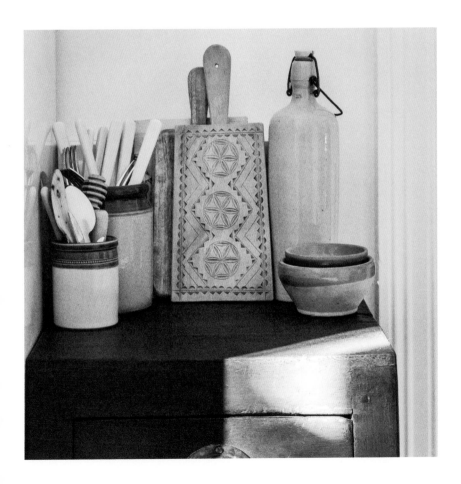

Decluttering Your Home

Here are some simple, tried-and-true tips for decluttering your home.

Pick one area to focus on. Don't try to tackle the whole house at once. Chances are you will feel overwhelmed and never actually begin.

Sort by category, not by room. This great tip from organizational guru Marie Kondo means you will not repeat the task over and over. It is also harder to decide what you can let go of when you haven't actually collected all the items together.

Organize your belongings. As soon as you have cleared the clutter, organize your things. Put like with like (e.g., all batteries together, all spare bedding in one place). In order to have a tidy home, every item needs a place to be tidied away into.

Utilize storage. It is amazing what good storage can do for a room; effective storage allows you to have less surface clutter. Make the most of the space you have, by using extra hooks or by storing things under your bed or sofa. Try to keep the contents of all storage and drawers tidy, too, so things are easy to find. If there are lots of smaller items in one drawer, subdivide the items into containers. Just be careful that you don't use the storage as an excuse to hoard more things.

Go digital. Can you go paperless with banking, paying bills, etc.? Or is it time to digitize all of your CDs?

Try to tidy little and often.
Things come in and out of our homes on a daily basis; therefore, it is important to tidy frequently. Make it part of your weekly routine to stay on top of the clutter by putting time aside—only fifteen minutes a day—to sort through it regularly. It's amazing the difference fifteen minutes a day can make.

Involve your children. Help your children learn from a young age where things live in your home. By teaching them the importance of putting things away, they will be able to help you keep your home tidy. It will also help them appreciate their toys and belongings, which is an important step in establishing healthy boundaries when shopping with your children.

Sort your paperwork.
Paperwork comes into most homes daily, in the form of letters, bills, notifications from school, etc. Think about setting up a system for how and where this paperwork can be stored, recycled, and shredded. This will help reduce paper clutter and also make it easier to find things.

Collect charity donations.
Have a bag for charity donations somewhere in your home. When you come across something that isn't used or needed, it can go straight into the bag. When the bag is full, donate it to the local charity shop.

Create a memory box. Designate a box for sentimental items that you want to keep but that don't necessarily need to be displayed in your home. We have created one especially for our daughter, as she often creates drawings and artwork, along with schoolwork, that we want to hold on to and treasure. By creating a memory box, you have somewhere specific to put those precious items, without them spreading throughout your home. Remember to be mindful about what you keep and place in the box.

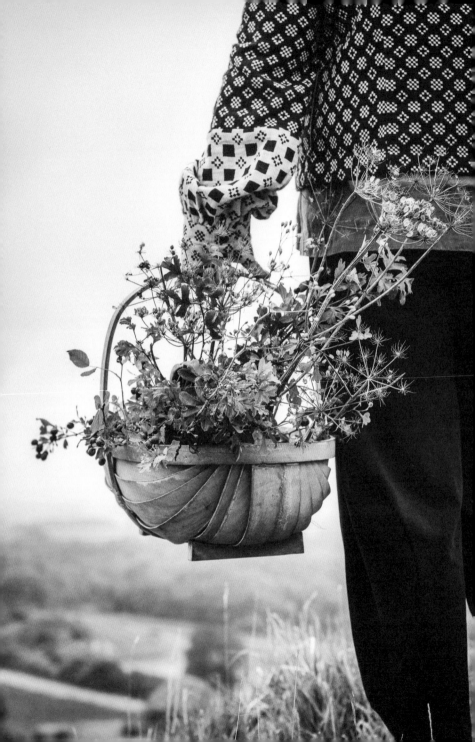

Seasonal
Living

....

Connecting to and understanding the seasons has been a big part of my family's slow-living journey. There is so much inspiration to be found in nature and the seasons with regard to slowing down and living more simply. Nature does not know how to hurry; the blossoms bloom when they are ready and the leaves fall when it is time. Living seasonally gives the year a shape and rhythm of its own and a lot of comfort can be gained from familiarity with these rhythms.

HOW TO LIVE SEASONALLY

Living seasonally is easy to do. We can start by observing what happens during each season within the natural world. What changes are happening with the weather? What is going on with wildlife? Go out into nature and the countryside and look at what is growing in the hedgerows and your local surroundings, such as what flowers are blooming. Even if you live in a city, there will be seasonal things to notice. By observing nature, including weather patterns, phases of the moon, and tide times, among other things, you will undoubtedly notice yourself responding to the seasons in a different way. You can also look at what seasonal festivals and traditions are happening each month.

By closely observing each season and what's happening outside our window, we can gain a greater connection to our immediate surroundings. It also encourages a natural affinity for the earth in general and fosters the desire to look after the land around us, and, of course, our planet. Feeling connected to something in this way is life-affirming. By embracing the differences of each season (and each month), we will find more joy in the simple things and will also be reminded how fleeting time can be.

WELCOMING THE SEASONS

In order to deepen our alignment with the seasons and nature, there are many simple things we can do. Visit a local farmers' market and buy the fruits and vegetables that are in season. In December, feast on chestnuts, cranberries, and clementines; in June, enjoy fresh cherries, strawberries, and summer squash.

Or look at what things you can do to support your well-being and your family's general health through the upcoming season. For example, rose hips are ready to be picked in late autumn; they are a great source of vitamin C and are considered a superfood because of how much good stuff they are packed with. You could try making a tea or syrup with them to help support and prepare your body and immune system for winter.

Finally, you can look to the seasons to inform how you use and decorate your space at home. By bringing nature into your home and using seasonal elements for displays and family activities, it reminds you of and connects you to the season, even when you're not outside. We love to bring seasonal elements into our home, and the process of collecting pieces of nature that represent that season has become a tradition and joyous act in itself. In autumn, we collect leaves and conkers for craft projects and bring gourds and pumpkins into our home for decoration. Autumn is also the time that I start to light candles around our home again, as the days begin to draw in and the early evening gets darker. Decorating your home with seasonal nature finds is such a simple thing to begin to do with your family.

Within nature and the seasons, there are so many inspiring and creative opportunities that are just waiting to be discovered. All you need to do is step outside, look around, and take a moment to notice.

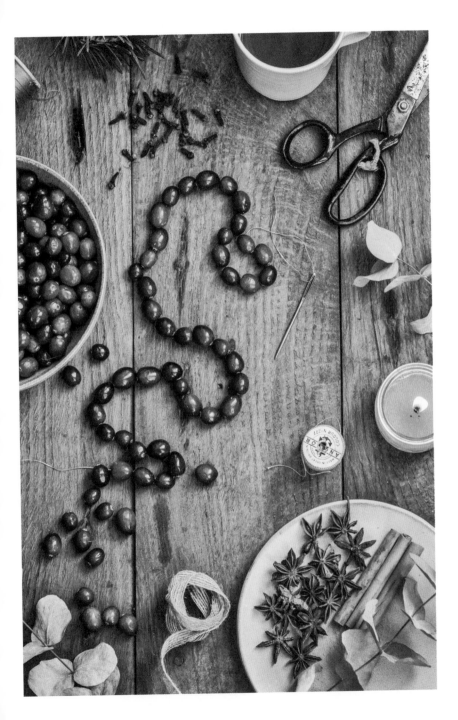

Seasonal Decorations and Activities

SPRING

Gathering blossom branches. Blossom might be the ultimate sign of spring, so bring blossom branches into your home.

Snowdrop spotting. Snowdrops are often called the "heralds of spring," so head out to see the first signs that winter is transitioning into spring.

Stick weaving. Weave twine through a forked stick and then weave in nature finds, such as leaves, flowers, and feathers.

Sounds of spring. Head deep into the countryside and listen for the sounds of spring, such as birdsong, the hum of buzzing bees, and lambs bleating.

Lambing. Go to a local farm to see the lambs being born.

SUMMER

Flower crowns. Weave a flower crown from foraged bits of flora and greenery.

Flower pressing. Collect local flowers to press, and then get creative with the pressings.

Beach mosaic (a wonderful activity to do with children). Create your own mosaic and pictures from things that you find on the beach, including shells, driftwood, seaweed, etc.

Nature boat (the perfect activity for an afternoon by the river or at rock pools at low tide). Make a boat from pieces of nature such as leaves, driftwood, twigs, etc.

Fairy house. Get creative and let your little ones build a fairy house in the woods for woodland fairies and elves.

Here are some ideas for seasonal decorations and activities to help you connect to what is happening in the natural world. The ideas for decorations to make often involve going out into nature to collect something seasonal for the creation, which are perfect activities for getting children outdoors and exploring. Why not try starting your own family seasonal traditions?

AUTUMN

Leaf garland. Gather leaves from an autumnal walk to string up at home.

Leaf crown. Get creative and make your own leaf crown, perfect for an autumn prince or princess.

Conker necklace. All you need is thread and conkers to make the perfect autumnal necklace.

Autumn art. Use the autumn leaves as inspiration and a starting point for children's artwork; there are many things you can make and create, from leaf animals to leaf rubbings and leaf confetti.

Leaf mandalas. Gather all the beautiful colors of autumn to create outdoor leaf mandalas.

WINTER

Winter wreath. Gather greenery to create your own winter wreath.

Homemade Advent calendar. There are many simple ways you can mark the passing of Advent.

Popcorn and cranberry garlands. Making homemade popcorn is such fun, and it's very easy to string together with cranberries for wonderful, natural Christmas decorations.

Orange slices. Bake orange slices to make into decorations to hang from the tree or make into a garland. This activity will also make your home smell gloriously festive.

Foraging for greenery. Go for a walk to forage for as much greenery as possible to decorate your home with.

NATURE THERAPY

Seasonal living and spending time in nature go hand in hand, and there is something about being out in the wilds of nature that can't be replicated by anything else. Writers, composers, and artists have been trying to capture the majesty of nature for centuries. And recently, the Japanese practice of *shinrin-yoku*, or forest bathing, has started to become more popular in Western culture.

Perhaps due to urbanization or the fact that many of us spend our days sitting behind a computer, there seems to be a resurgence of people wanting to reconnect to nature.[12] Many of us are realizing that spending time in nature has a positive impact on our well-being. Nature therapy, also known as ecotherapy, helps a person in a stressed state by using the restorative effect of nature for physiological relaxation.[13] By spending time outside in fresh air, reconnecting to the wilds of nature, we begin to feel relaxed and calm. Research is being done all the time into the regenerative properties of being close to nature and how it can help improve mood and alleviate depression and anxiety, and nature therapy is becoming increasingly popular with mental health-care professionals. Some health-care professionals are even issuing "nature prescriptions" for medical conditions, such as high blood pressure and diabetes.

Time outdoors in a big expanse of nature can't but help put any problem into perspective. It reminds us that

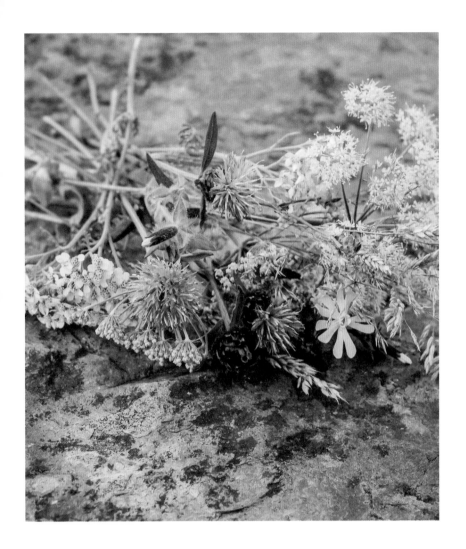

we are all part of something greater and bigger than ourselves. By acknowledging that time spent in nature grounds us and enhances our well-being, we are also reminded to enjoy the nature that is around us as much as possible.

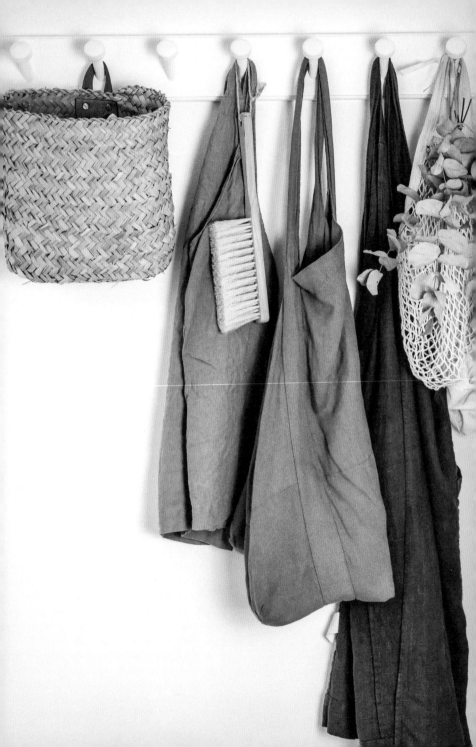

Sustainability

....

When slowing our homes, we also need to consider reducing our environmental impact. There
are two key areas to examine to live as sustainably
as possible: our conscious shopping habits (this
applies to everything from shopping for food,
housewares, and clothing to luxuries and cleaning
and beauty products) and how responsible we are
when disposing of any waste we create.

CONSCIOUS SHOPPING

Once we have gone to all the hard work of decluttering, we don't want to fill our homes with "stuff" again. We can drastically reduce how much we consume if we buy less and choose well. Buying low-cost things that aren't well made is a false economy (where we think we are saving money, but actually, we end up spending more because the items need replacing more frequently). Along with affecting our expenses, these choices also impact the resources of the planet. When we understand that resources are finite and that our actions have consequences, for everyone and our planet's well-being, the context of how we buy things is suddenly very different, and of course influences the choices we make as consumers. When shopping, there are some helpful questions that you can ask yourself when considering a purchase:

» **Do I really need this item?**

» **Do I need to buy it new, or can I buy or source it some other way (secondhand/vintage/antique)?**

» **Is the item well made and will it last?**

» **Do I know where and how this item was made? Is it ethical?**

» **What is its environmental impact?**

» How is this item packaged? Is there a lot of extra packaging that this product doesn't need? Can I buy an alternative that creates less waste?

SLOW FASHION

When it comes to our wardrobes, it seems that a buy-and-throw-away attitude has become more prevalent because of the proliferation of fast fashion options. Since 2000, clothing sales have approximately doubled, whereas the number of times we wear an item of clothing has decreased significantly.[14] "Slow fashion" is a term that was conceived in 2008 by sustainable-design consultant Kate Fletcher. She wanted to address the speed of the entire fashion cycle, as well as look at how environmentally friendly the production of a single item of clothing is.

The rapid consumption of clothing created by fast-fashion retailers and the carbon-intensive supply chains and production processes result in the fashion industry's carbon emissions being greater than the international aviation and maritime industries combined.[15] We have come to expect to pay a certain price for mass-produced clothing, but with the spotlight being shone on the workings of the fashion industry, now is the time to stop and question the true cost of low-priced clothes.

Originally, there were two fashion collections a year: autumn/winter and spring/summer. Through the onset of "fast fashion" and the ability to quickly and cheaply copy catwalk looks, lots of high-end fashion labels have increased their number of collections in order to stay one step ahead. Some fast fashion brands have also added "micro seasons,"[16] and there can be as many as fifty-two collections a year, meaning there can be something new to entice us into their shops every week. Collections have only increased because there is the appetite to consume more.

Society will always be interested in fashion, partly because nothing expresses our identity as much as the clothes we wear, but we are beginning to realize that we cannot continue to consume fashion at this pace. Most of us are aware that there is a problem with textile waste, with the majority of clothing ending up in landfills within the first year of being purchased. However, a lot of the damage is happening at the beginning of the supply chain, from how we grow and harvest fibers to the water and chemical footprint and dye pollution.[17] Also, social sustainability is a big concern. Most of our clothes are made overseas with 97 percent of production being sourced to developing countries. Who is making our clothes? Are they paid fairly? What are their working conditions like? According to Global Fashion Agenda, "Over 50 percent of workers are not paid the minimum wage in countries like India and the Philippines."[18]

It's our responsibility as consumers to become more conscious about what we buy, the fashion supply chain, and how something is made. We need to ask the important questions, like "How can this piece of clothing be made at such a low cost?" and "Do I really need another pair of shoes?" Trying to choose items that have minimum impact on the environment can be a challenge, especially if things aren't clearly labeled, and may be beyond our budgets; however, there are practical things we can do to join the slow fashion movement and reduce our clothing consumption.

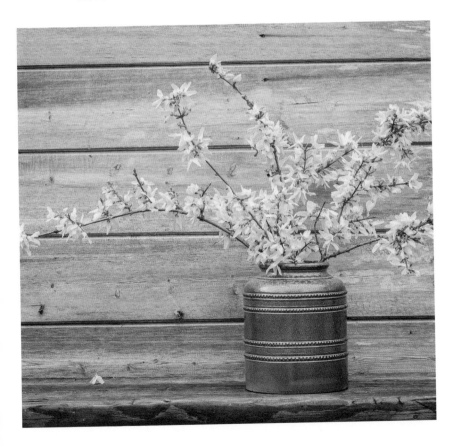

Conscious Consumerism

By shifting our thinking and by making a few small changes we can reduce our impact on the planet through the consumer choices we make. Here are some simple ideas to help you become a more conscious consumer.

Buy less and choose well. By referring to the phrases "buy less and choose well" and "quality over quantity," we can aim to buy things that are well made and therefore will last longer. It is also helpful to think about the longevity of an item and buy timeless pieces that you will be able to use over and over again. If we invest in trend-driven items, we are more likely to not like an item when it goes out of style.

Buy secondhand and vintage. This is a good environmentally friendly option, especially for clothes and furniture, as the carbon footprint is a lot less than a newly made item. With so many great charity shops and thrift stores, you can get most items secondhand now, from books and children's clothes to crockery and DVDs.

Get the most out of what you already own. Try to take extra-special care of your belongings and really wear out things. You will find that you automatically buy less when making the most out of the items you have. Once clothes and shoes are worn, or if items get damaged, they can be repaired or recycled.

Cherish inherited items. Hand-me-downs and inherited objects from friends and family are a great way to reuse items. We have lots of inherited items in our home, particularly where furniture is concerned. I love that we have my husband's great-grandmother's Ercol chair and that we have a bureau that used to belong to my great-grandmother. It's these items that personalize our home and give it character.

Be mindful when shopping for growing children. Remember to be mindful about how many toys we buy for our children—they don't need as much as we think they do. Toys, clothes, and books can be passed on to friends or donated to charity when they have been outgrown. In terms of clothing for children, it can be challenging shopping for a growing child and buying items of clothing that will last. Try to always look for simple shapes and buy a size up when possible. Items that are originally dresses can later be worn as tunics or long tops.

Look for ethical labels. Do research and look at how an item is labeled to help identify how ethical a product is. Depending on your purchase, look for accredited labels, including fair trade, organic, cruelty-free, vegan, etc. Regarding beauty and skincare products, if you are unsure, look at the listed ingredients.

Think about packaging and reduce your use of single-use plastics. Single-use plastics include straws, food packaging, drink bottles, and takeout coffee cups, lids, and stirrers. There are simple alternatives that are easy to implement, such as paper straws, reusable drink bottles, and reusable coffee cups. Gradually, countries are reducing and banning the use of plastic bags, so get in the habit of bringing your own reusable bags for grocery shopping. Try to buy fruit and vegetables that aren't packaged in anything. If your local supermarket is still packaging items, shop at your local independent grocery store or farmers market. For bagging individual fruit and vegetables items, you can buy reusable muslin fabric bags.

Try to shop locally. Shopping locally helps reinvigorate your local community. Often, local independent retailers support other local business, keeping the supply chain local.

Remember that your consumer choices have power. By consciously deciding what you want to spend your money on, you are effectively voting with your wallet. You have the power to boycott companies and products that aren't being responsible or ethical. And you also have the power to support companies and shops that give back by donating money to good causes.

REDUCE, REUSE, RECYCLE

It makes sense that by reducing what we consume, we will automatically reduce our waste too. Once we have cut back on our consumption as much as possible, it's good to make sure that any waste we create is disposed of in the most environmentally friendly way.

It is natural to feel a bit daunted when looking at things like environmentalism and reducing our waste. In fact, even the term "zero waste" feels unattainable for many. Because the problems we are facing are so extreme and complex, it is easy to feel like there is a right and a wrong way to do things, which can leave us confused about where to start. However, the little things we do as individuals can add up to make a big difference, and we can be empowered by the small daily changes we can make. When looking at reducing our waste and sustainability, it is important that we ensure that any changes we make are not only sustainable for the planet but for our lifestyles too. In fact, we are more likely to stay motivated and maintain any adjustments by taking manageable steps.

Recycling. Recycling is the first, easy step we can take to sustainably reduce our waste. In fact, most communities have mandated recycling programs in place and will even fine those in the United States who do not abide by the rules and procedures. Still, these recycling programs don't take care of everything, leaving a lot of packaging that ends up in the regular trash and therefore in landfill. However, a lot of these items can be recycled too. By looking farther afield than our normal refuse collection, many of us will find that there are additional local projects available to help us recycle more. If you are not sure where to begin with your recycling, you could start by sorting through your weekly trash to see which items appear time and time again. Then you will be able to target a specific sort of packaging and find the best way to recycle it.

Food waste. How we dispose of our food waste is an easy way to reduce our overall waste. Firstly, take some time to make clever choices about the food you buy and what you cook to avoid excessive waste. For example, try a weekly meal plan and factor in leftovers, etc. If we throw our food waste in with our general rubbish, it rots in landfill and creates methane, a damaging greenhouse gas. By separating our food waste, we can dispose of it safely and help create useful by-products, such as soil improver and fertilizer, and even generate electricity. There are several different options for separating out food waste depending on one's circumstances. Compost bins are a great way to get rid of your food waste if you have space in your garden. However, if setting up your own compost seems like a step too far, see if there is community composting. If you have a small garden or live in an apartment, you could try disposing of your food waste using a wormery (worm farm) or a bokashi bin for composting. There are also other alternatives, and they all have their good points and compromises, so spend some time doing your own research in order to make sure you choose something that will work for you and will be sustainable.

Reuse and restore. Another way to make our resources go further is to reuse and restore things. It is very satisfying to be able to use things to their full potential. If we can learn to take extra-special care of our things, they will last longer; when they do finally wear out, we need to think about how and whether they can be mended, and if they can't, perhaps they can be reused or repurposed as something else. These principles can be applied to all areas of our lives, from clothing and furniture to general household items. This "make do and mend" mind-set is nothing new. Generations before us were often thrifty with their possessions out of necessity. This thinking also encourages us to acquire the skills to be more self-sufficient. Having a DIY approach to fixing, restoring, or making something ourselves is a great alternative to buying something new. Even though it takes an investment in time and energy, it means we can make exactly what we want to our specific requirements, and we end up with something bespoke. Also, this process becomes a labor of love—we will naturally end up cherishing and appreciating the finished result through the investment of time and effort.

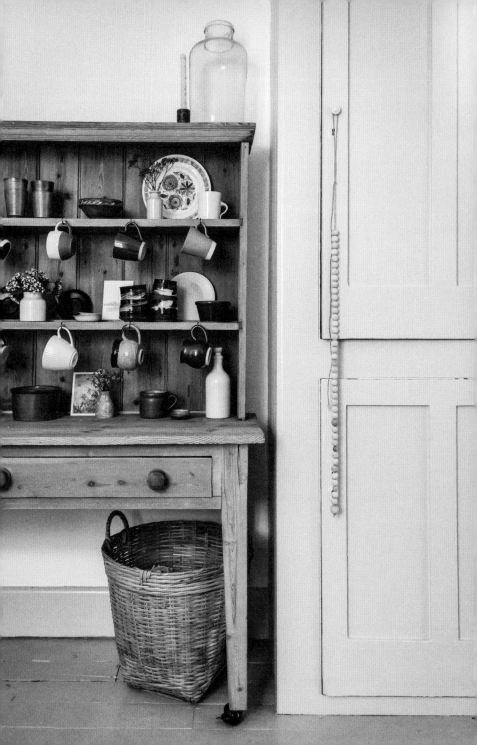

A HOMEGROWN AND NATURAL HOME

There are many benefits to having a homegrown home. Along with saving money and cultivating truly organic food, which is better for our health, growing our own produce reduces our impact on the planet because less resources are used. There is no transportation from grower to manufacturer to shop, and of course, we cut down on any packaging waste.

You don't need a big garden to start growing your own food. Lots of things can be grown in pots and grow bags. Some easy crops to try to begin with are lettuces, cucumbers, and tomatoes. Zucchini is also a good vegetable to start with, although you do need a bit more space for it. If growing things from seed seems a little daunting, you can always start from a seedling, which you can buy from your local garden center or nursery, or even initiate a plant swap within your local community.

If you aren't ready to commit to a homegrown home, a natural home is easy to attain. Think about the products you use to clean and run your home, and the cleansing and beauty products you and your family use. How natural are they? How good are they for your health and well-being? Do they contain chemicals that are harmful to your body and the planet?

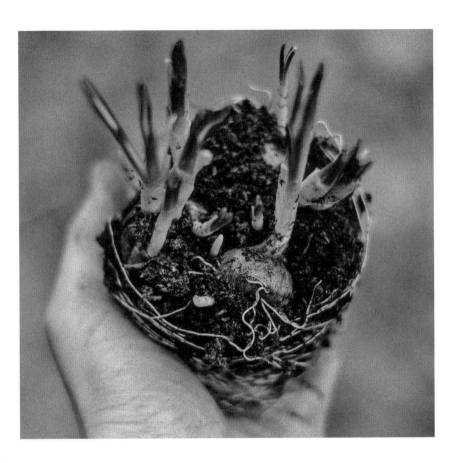

Fortunately, there are more and more products available that are natural and chemical-free. Also, you could try making your own products, so you are aware of the exact ingredients. Plus, doing this will drastically cut down on packaging waste, because you can reuse the containers over and over.

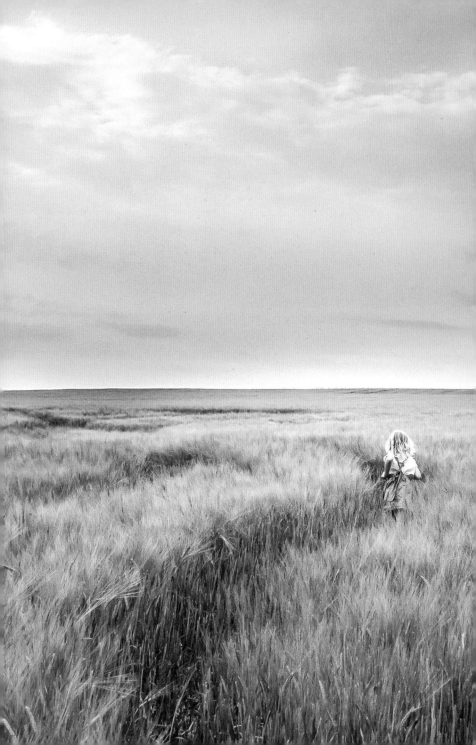

Well-Being

MIND AND SOUL

....

When we begin to live more slowly, we find we have time to look within—space unfolds and allows us to deeply think and reevaluate things. We have time to think about the purpose and meaning within our lives, and naturally, we become more intentional and thoughtful with the decisions we make. Both meditation and mindfulness are explorations of the mind and help us be more thoughtful, focused, and calm. Practicing meditation and mindfulness is the perfect way to take the time to understand the intricacies of our minds and ourselves. They can bring out the best side of human nature and help us cope with the day-to-day challenges that life throws at us, like stress at work, paying our bills, and raising children.

WHAT IS MEDITATION?

I have talked a lot in this book about "being in the present moment," and meditation is a way to help us truly experience what being in the present feels like. "Being in the present moment" means not being distracted by the past and not worrying about the future—just being in the now and experiencing what is right in front of us. As we become more capable of doing this, we can then try to be present in that moment without judgment or attachment.

Meditation encompasses a wide range of practices at different levels, from the advanced techniques that yogis and monks have practiced for centuries to mindfulness techniques (exercises that help you focus on something specific about the present moment) and meditation apps. The practice of meditation has accelerated since the late 1960s, as interest has increased in Western culture. Along with this proliferation, the meaning of the word has also evolved. Traditional meditation techniques have gradually been developed and watered down in order to make meditation and its benefits as accessible as possible.

In its purest form, meditation gives us a better understanding of ourselves and our true natures; it essentially helps us to discover who we are. As human beings, it is natural to be longing and searching for meaning and purpose within our lives, and meditation can help us delve into the depths of these internal discussions. The philosophical nature of these questions and ideas means that meditation often feels connected to a spiritual practice and discovery. However, regardless of one's spiritual or religious beliefs, such philosophical thinking can be hard to ignore, and most of us at some point or another realize it is important to explore such fundamental questions.

Throughout history, meditation has been connected to many religions, including Buddhism, Hinduism, Sikhism, and even Christianity; however, meditation can be practiced by anyone regardless of their faith. Due to the wide variety of techniques available today, we can select the aspects of meditation that interest and inspire us.

WHAT IS MINDFULNESS?

Mindfulness is a wakeful awareness that encourages us to train our attention and it has become an increasingly popular practice. The term "mindfulness" originates from a rough translation of the Buddhist word *sati*, which is the first factor of the seven factors of enlightenment in Buddhism. Over the last forty years, the dissemination of mindfulness has resulted in its meaning becoming muddied. Currently, mindfulness encompasses MBSR (mindfulness-based stress reduction), MBCT (mindfulness-based cognitive therapy), Vipassana (a Theravada Buddhism meditation that cultivates awareness), a stop-and-smell-the-roses attitude, and a lifestyle trend.

Perhaps the term "mindfulness" has become popular because it feels accessible, partly due to the impression that it is a secular practice. People also find it easy to see how they would be able to slot mindfulness into their current lifestyle. There are many mindfulness techniques that encourage you to focus on one specific aspect of the present moment, such as the raisin exercise, where you take your time to intentionally, hold, see, smell, and consciously eat one raisin, or the body scan exercise, where you scan your body from head to toe focusing on each individual part in detail. Practically, you can bring a mindful approach and your focused attention to any daily task. In reality, because mindfulness has roots in meditation, many of its aims, techniques, and approaches are similar.

WHY MEDITATE AND PRACTICE MINDFULNESS?

Meditation is like hitting a reset button each day. Any challenges or difficulties that have arisen over the last twenty-four hours float to the surface and dissipate. Meditation allows us the space to return to a neutral mind, helping us to not become fixated on or attached to negative thoughts and emotions. Meditation also helps us be aware of the tension our bodies can hold. By sitting and focusing on our breath for extended periods of time, we notice parts of our bodies awaken with the flow of breath and energy as we begin to let go of any tension. Learning to be present in the moment helps when challenging situations arise; we find that we don't have an emotional knee-jerk reaction but are able to take a moment to mindfully react, so generally we are able to remain calm and act with more compassion.

One main principle behind meditation is to calm our minds, which are often full of thoughts and internal chatter. An analogy of a lake is often used to help explain why a calm mind is so important. Imagine that our thoughts are like the water: A busy, restless mind equals a choppy lake in which the water turns murky due to the bottom of the lake being disturbed. It is then impossible to see below the surface. However, when the lake is calm and still, the water is clear and you can see with clarity down to the depths of the lake bed. In order to know our true selves, we have to learn to look within, and we can only do this once we have learned how to still the mind and quiet the chatter.

Both mindfulness and meditation can and have been used to provide therapeutic benefit to reduce things like stress and anxiety, and help with depression. "In a meta-analysis of forty-seven studies on the application of meditation methods to treat patients with mental health problems, the findings show that meditation can lead to decreases in depression (particularly severe depression), anxiety and pain."[19]

Along with producing general feelings of well-being and peace, meditation also has the potential, with a regular, in-depth practice, to change character traits and habits. As previously mentioned, there are different levels of meditation, so the benefits will vary depending on your practice. How long you sit and meditate for, how regularly, and how you progress with the meditation will all have an effect on the outcome. A day retreat will provide a temporary oasis in altered states, but to make long-lasting changes, you will need to commit to a regular practice. "After continued practice, we notice some changes in our way of being, but they come and go. Finally, as practice stabilizes, the changes are constant and enduring, with no fluctuation. They are altered traits."[20]

The Benefits of Meditation

Even though meditation is a practice of the mind, it affects our whole being—physical, mental, emotional and spiritual. Here are some of the benefits of doing it.

Cultivates mindful awareness

Relieves stress and tension

Brings a sense of peace

Rejuvenates the mind

Deepens our sense of focus

Allows us to feel more present

Expands consciousness

Helps us get a more restful night's sleep

Helps us connect to our inner selves

Develops our understanding and control of our breath and prana (energy)

Enhances feelings of well-being

Creates detachment from our emotions (less bothered by the little things)

MEDITATION TECHNIQUES

There are lots of different types of meditation. When starting out as a beginner, it can be helpful to decide whether you want to try a guided meditation, in which you follow a voice instructing you with a specific focus, task, or visualization, or whether you want to try to meditate independently.

Some examples of guided meditation are body-scanning meditation, breath-awareness meditation, and loving-kindness meditation. Some examples of independent meditation are transcendental meditation, mindfulness meditations, and moving meditation.

Most types of meditation can fall within both the guided and independent practices; however, practicing a guided meditation and meditating in solitude are very different experiences. Both have their positives aspects and challenges, and by trying each type, you will be able to ascertain when to use which practice.

Remember that to begin with, just creating the space for your practice and sitting with the intention is the hardest part. Nearly all meditators, regardless of the specific practice, are undertaking the process of main-taining their focus. They notice the mind wandering and gently bring it back to whatever their focus is, be it a mantra, a breath pattern, or a visual point.

HOW TO BEGIN TO MEDITATE

If you are new to meditation, it is normal to feel a little overwhelmed by the prospect of learning to meditate. You might wonder how and where to start, and whether you are meditating properly. A good starting point is to choose a meditation that appeals to you and stick with it consistently for a realistic amount of time each day. The repetition of a daily practice is important and consistency is key (see Daily Slow-Living Rituals on page 113).

Take comfort in the fact that many people find meditation challenging in the beginning, especially if you have a very active mind—just sitting in stillness can be excruciatingly difficult. In this case, moving meditation and mantras can be helpful. The repetitive movement and/or the repetitive mantra give the mind something concrete to focus on and a tangible task to channel any excess energy into. Focusing on "emptying your mind" is almost impossible; it is like being told not to think of a white bear,[21] which of course guarantees that you will think only of white bears. Instead, when meditating, try to find those moments of stillness and stay present in them.

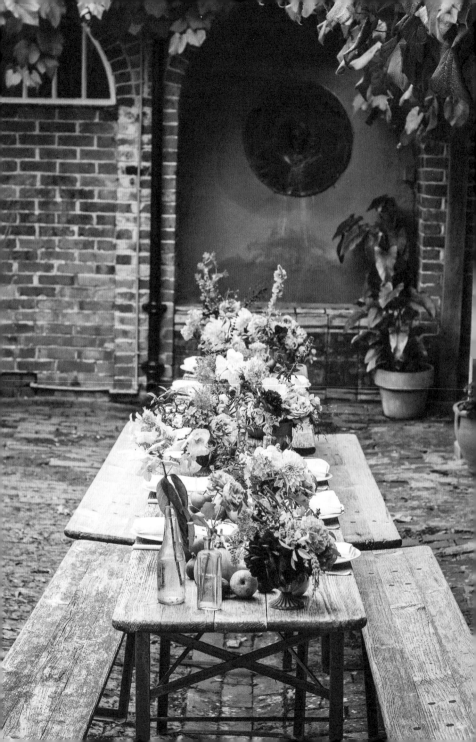

Daily Slow-Living Rituals

....

There is an art to creating a ritual. A ritual is a moment that we consciously take the time to absorb and be truly present in. If we deconstruct it, a ritual is a ceremony of a series of sacred actions. Tiu De Haan, ritual designer and inspirational speaker, describes a ritual as a container around a moment, rather like a frame around a piece of art. She also explains that a "ritual nourishes the soul like food and water nourish the body."[22] Rituals can bring moments of reverence into our days in the simplest ways. The art of the ritual becomes a visual and physical cue for our body to slow down, be mindful, breathe a little deeper, and be more present. By understanding a ritual in these terms, we can see the benefit of making rituals a part of our daily routine.

CREATING A RITUAL

There are simple daily tasks we already do that have the potential to become a ritual—things like making a cup of tea or washing our hands; everyday activities that we might otherwise consider mundane can in fact be cherished and completed in a conscious way. By setting a clear intention with how we perform the task, we can use the everyday ritual as a way to connect to ourselves and slow down. Let's take the example of making a cup of tea: In some cultures, this act is indeed a beautiful and lengthy ritual that is done with a lot of reverence. We don't need to go as far as performing a Japanese tea ceremony to make our morning cup of tea, but there is something to be learned from this mindful and thoughtful tradition. By really observing each detail of the activity, we absorb ourselves in the task in front of us and allow our mind and body to slow down and find a little quiet during the process.

We can consciously turn our slow moments (see page 52), which we uncovered earlier, into rituals. Rather than just letting them pass us by, we can create a ceremony out of many everyday pleasures. It only takes a little bit of thought and creativity to turn any slow moment into a ritual. You can create a ritual by linking a few moments together, or by focusing in on the simple joy of a task, or by amplifying sections of the activity and adorning and embellishing them. These moments, when consciously turned into rituals, can be important signifiers for your body, mind, and soul that you are moving from one type of task and energy into a slow and calm mind-set. For example, if you work from home, you could try creating a mini ritual of lighting a candle to mark the end of the working day. Or you could establish a gardening ritual, where you walk around your garden and tend to it for ten minutes to help you switch off and shut down the working part of your day and welcome your evening in a relaxed manner.

Along with slow-living rituals, there are also a wealth of complementary well-being practices that you can integrate as rituals into your life in order to live more holistically—meditation, mindfulness, yoga, self-massage, etc. Adding any of these to your wellness repertoire can be a great way to reconnect with yourself.

FROM RITUAL, TO ROUTINE, TO HABIT

Although a ritual is a special moment in itself, the repetition of any well-being ritual helps us begin to form new routines and, eventually, healthy habits. Through regularly performing the rituals, they gradually become part of our weekly routine. When something has been woven into a routine for a month or so, it then settles into a regular tendency, eventually becoming a habit.

Through the repetition of routine, our minds and bodies learn and relearn, and eventually, the routine becomes instinctive to us. This is the same process implemented by an athlete, a musician, or a dancer, who practices over and over until it is embedded in their muscle memory—this fine-tunes their motor skills, allowing them to perform the movement so automatically that it is effortless, and they don't have to consciously think about what they are doing.

If we want these new rituals to become a habit, then we will have to commit to them with consistency. In Kundalini yoga, it is said that it takes forty days to break a habit. The number forty holds great significance across lots of spiritual practices: Moses spent forty days on Mount Sinai, Christians fast for forty days for Lent, and Buddha meditated for forty days under the bodhi tree. Forty days isn't very long in the scheme of things; after all, we are talking about altering our routines, behaviors, and habits, so there are no quick fixes. It takes at least forty days of constant repetition to begin to retrain our thought patterns and nervous system. Then of course it takes even longer than forty days to establish that new habit, and make it instinctual to us.

The ideal situation is that, eventually, any slow-living rituals and well-being practices we do become deeply intertwined with our lifestyles and schedules. We don't want to have to remember to get our yoga mat out, or to breathe deeply, or to take some time to slow things down. We want them to be a natural and integrated part of our lives.

Daily Mindfulness

Pick an ordinary everyday activity. It could be preparing dinner, washing your hands or face, or hanging the laundry on the line.

Can you try to do the task mindfully? Can you bring your focus to all the little details of the activity? Think about the sounds you can hear, what smells you can notice, what textures you can feel.

Using the example of washing your hands, take the time to notice what the water feels like on your skin—the sensation, the temperature—the sound the water makes, the smell of the soap, how soft the towel feels when drying your hands.

Really engage all five senses to bring your attention to focus on the present moment that is right in front of you. If you find your mind wandering, gently bring it back to the task you are doing.

What did you notice?
How hard did you find this exercise?

ESTABLISHING A QUIET CORNER

It is important to have an area in our homes where we can relax, feel calm, and be at peace. Maybe you already have a handful of places you can retreat to in your home when life gets hectic, but if you live in a busy family home, trying to find space and time to sit and practice a breath exercise or meditation can be tricky.

It can be helpful to spend a little time thinking about how to create a calm space just for you, and where in your home you could create such a space. Having a designated space that is free from distractions can really help the mind settle down and stay focused. In fact, by regularly meditating in the same place, you can begin to infuse that corner of your home with a calm energy. You will probably notice that you start to breathe a little deeper by simply stepping onto your mat (before you even begin your practice).

Think of the best room in your house where you would be able to retreat to and get fifteen minutes of peace and quiet—perhaps your bedroom, spare room, or living room. Once you have chosen the room, decide where in the room you can create a calm space. There might be an obvious corner that lends itself for you to be able to do a simple meditation—you don't need a lot of space; an area about the size of a yoga mat is ideal. When deciding on the perfect spot for your

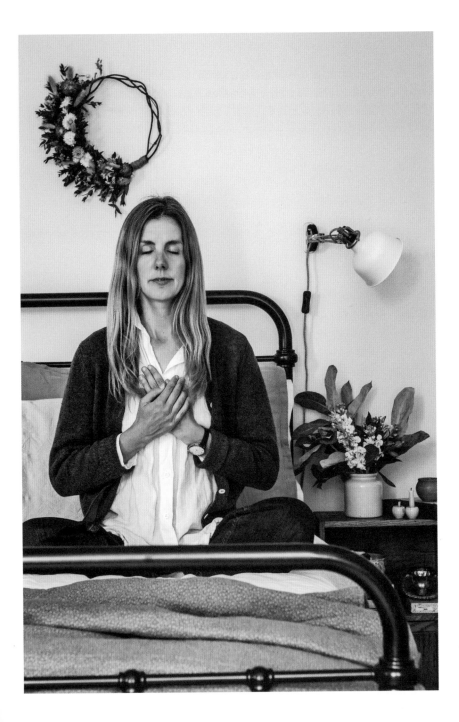

practice, you might also want to think about when you will be able to craft your fifteen minutes of quiet, which corner of the room gets the best light, etc. By creating this calm space, it naturally focuses your thoughts and clarifies your intention—notice the difference this process makes to your motivation and frame of mind.

Ideally, this will be a consistent space; however, if that is impossible, you can create a pop-up calm space that you can set up and put away as necessary. The setting up of your calm space will then become part of your practice. Rolling out the mat, lighting a candle, and burning a sage smudge stick are all part of the ritual, and become the signifier that you are about to turn your attention inward. These small acts of preparing the space will help get your mind and body ready for the practice too. Here are some items that can help you create that designated calm space at home:

» **Yoga mat**

» **Sheepskin**

» **Candles**

» **Smudge stick**

» **Crystals**

» **Relaxing music**

» **Yoga videos**

» **Online meditation apps, such as Insight Timer, Headspace, and Calm**

Once you have created one area like this inside your home, think about how elements of this area can filter through to other rooms of your home. This will help make your home as slow and calm as possible.

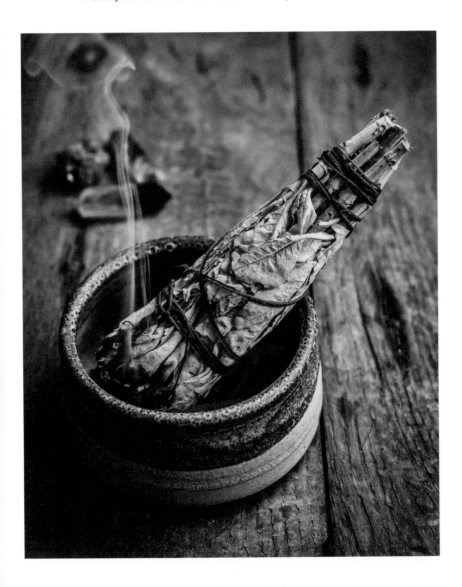

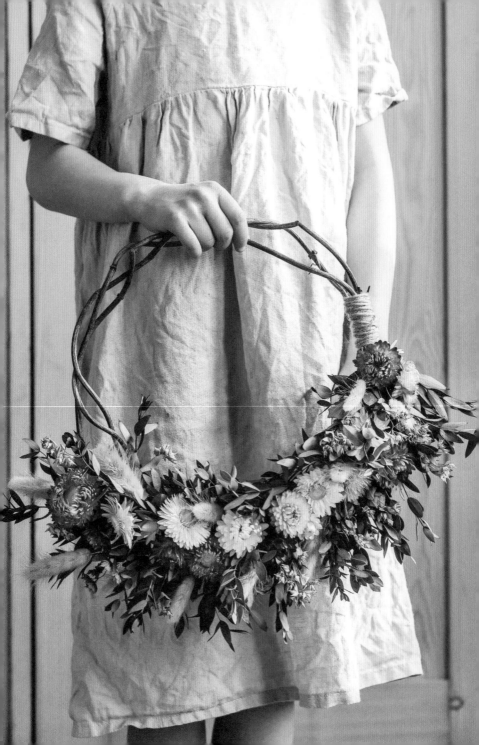

CONCLUSION

Throughout the past five years, my family has adapted many aspects of our lifestyle and altered our approach to how we schedule our weeks and prioritize our well-being. There is something inherent within us that knows that slowing down just makes sense, and I have seen time and time again how slow and simple living resonates with people.

More and more, I appreciate that time is the real luxury of life today—time to spend with loved ones and time to sit in moments of stillness. By slowing down, we are able to think about the purpose and meaning in our lives, and it's then that we realize that our well-being, and how happy and healthy we are, is what is most important. Once we start to think of time as a commodity, we naturally become more intentional with how we spend our time.

A large part of my family's slow-living experience has been the process of simplifying our home and our belongings. Our old house needs a lot of restoring and renovating, and uncovering the bare bones of this building has been a privilege, and has taught us a lot about the beauty and imperfection that can be added to something from the passing of time. It has also highlighted how crucial having patience is, especially when it comes to the timing of things, and that the art of waiting can indeed be a gift.

Living lightly is a work in progress, as we are constantly learning how to be more ethical. By analyzing our consumer culture, we have been able to make more conscious choices, address how much we consume, and be responsible for any waste we create.

Personally, I am finding that I crave more and more quiet time for my mind. I have learned that it's imperative to have space to play and daydream for my mental well-being, and I find that mindfully engaging in everyday tasks helps me stay present and grounded. On days and weeks when we are busy, I remember to value my slow moments and use them to create little punctuation marks in my day that allow me to pause and breathe a little deeper. As someone who works from home, I find that the daily slow-living rituals I have established are so important, because they act as little signifiers that I am switching pace, slowing down, and moving into a calm and nurturing space.

The further we look into simplifying our lives, the more I want distance from the digital age that we live in. Taking complete breaks from being at a computer or any sort of screen is what I have found works best for me. I have also found that I need to take breaks from social networks, too, especially as someone who is naturally a bit of an introvert. Being socially engaged all the time is tiring. With regular breaks, and my notifications switched off, I can intentionally choose when I am online, and that way I can be present and engaged. Having clear boundaries is only going to become more essential as technology continues to develop and becomes even more entwined with our lifestyles.

As a balance to this, we need to take comfort and find inspiration in nature. For my family, being in nature and connecting to the seasons continue to enrich our lives in new ways. I am constantly reminded how living seasonally can guide us and help us create healthy, authentic rhythms. I always turn to nature when things become challenging and it astounds me what a positive impact it has on my well-being.

If we want to start feeling happier and healthier, we have to reconnect and learn to listen to our bodies and remember that self-compassion is pivotal in slowing down and nurturing ourselves. We need to foster thoughtfulness and get to know our minds and ourselves inside out. Self-compassion is what I have been digging into recently. It's pretty fundamental to be able to relate to ourselves in a compassionate way, and for me, this is now key in order to deepen our slow-living experience. I know it will change the way I communicate with myself and the way I relate to those closest to me.

There are days where I still find it a challenge to be compassionate with myself and surrender to what my body needs. Maybe I have planned to do certain things, but when it comes to it, perhaps I simply don't have the energy; therefore, it makes sense to factor in more time to rest.

Understanding our bodies can be a challenge because they are constantly evolving. As I enter different seasons of my life, I find that I need different things to nourish and support my well-being. And equally, as my daughter grows, she requires different support and provides different challenges. We therefore have to remember to think about our well-being holistically and encourage ourselves to adapt. What continues to be a constant, though, is that inquisitive nature to understand myself and life a little better.

When it comes to altering our lifestyle and slowing down and simplifying, small daily changes can be empowering and help us feel like we are moving in the right direction. Sometimes, these simple realizations are all that are needed to initiate change, and by making small adjustments, we can begin to notice a difference in the quality of how we move through our weeks.

Once we start to think of our lives in terms of how happy and healthy we are, slow living naturally follows suit. After a while, we realize it simply makes sense to live this way and it feels like returning to a more authentic way to live. By living slowly and simply, we can create more space for quiet pauses and moments of stillness. The deeper understanding we have of ourselves, the more we are able to shape our future into what we really want. Let's honor our bodies and develop the art of listening to what we really need, not just the louder messages but the whispers from the soul as well.

ACKNOWLEDGMENTS

THANK YOU to Leo and Bailey for all the words of encouragement and extra huggles—I couldn't have got to this point without you. Your patience and help with taking pictures is invaluable. Thanks for always giving me the space to stop and capture what inspires me.

Thanks to my folks for raising me with an appreciation of the simple things, and for always encouraging me to do what makes me happy.

Many thanks to everyone who has listened and offered support whilst I have been thoroughly absorbed in creating this book—I promise I will start behaving normally again soon. Thanks to Sarah-Lou for taking a wonderful headshot (that I actually like) and for always listening.

Thanks to Rage for giving me the opportunity to share what slow living means to me and my family, to Erin for all your hard work with editing the book and for always answering my many emails, and to all those at Rock Point publishing that have worked so hard to help me make this book beautiful.

Thanks to everyone who reads my blog, subscribes to the newsletter, and follows along with our slow living journey. I hope this book inspires you to seek your own slice of slow.

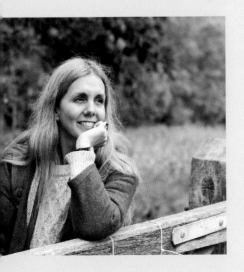

ABOUT THE AUTHOR

MELANIE BARNES is the writer and photographer behind the blog *Geoffrey and Grace* and the Instagram @geoffreyandgrace—destinations for slow and simple living. With more than fifteen years' experience in movement and well-being, she is a trained yogi, meditation teacher, and massage therapist. She shares advice on slow and simple living via her blog, e-guides, slow-living retreats, and magazine articles. She lives by the sea in Sussex in the UK with her husband, daughter, and cat.

NOTES

THE CHALLENGES OF OUR MODERN AGE

1. Professor Hollie Martin, "Consumer Culture/Materialism," YouTube, 2014.

2. Paulina Pchelin and Ryan T. Howell, "The Hidden Cost of Value-Seeking: People Do Not Accurately Forecast the Economic Benefits of Experiential Purchases," *The Journal of Positive Psychology*, 9 (2014): 322–34.

TIME

3. Daniel J. Levitin, *The Organized Mind: Thinking Straight in the Age of Information Overload* (New York: Plume, 2014), 16

4. Ibid., 96.

5. Ibid., 98.

LEARNING TO NURTURE OURSELVES

6. Kristin Neff, PhD, and Christopher Germer, PhD, *The Mindful Self-Compassion Workbook: A Proven Way to Accept Yourself, Build Inner Strength, and Thrive* (New York: The Guilford Press, 2018), 10.

7. Ibid., 1.

8. Dr. Stuart Brown, "Play Is More Than Just Fun," TED, 2008.

9. Indre Viskontas, "How Daydreaming Can Fix Your Brain," *Mother Jones* online, October 13, 2014.

10. Daniel J. Levitin, *The Organized Mind* (New York: Plume, 2014), 376.

11. Ibid., 170.

SEASONAL LIVING

12. Chorong Song, Harumi Ikei, and Yoshifumi Miyazaki, "Physiological Effects of Nature Therapy: A Review of the Research in Japan," *International Journal of Environmental Research and Public Health*, 13 (2016): 781.

13. Ibid.

SUSTAINABILITY

14. Ellen MacArthur Foundation, "A New Textiles Economy: Redesigning Fashion's Future" (Cowes: Ellen MacArthur Foundation, 2017), 18.

15. Ibid., 3.

16. Shannon Whitehead Lohr, "5 Truths the Fashion Industry Doesn't Want You to Know" *Life* (blog), HuffPost, October 19, 2014 (updated).

17. Ellen MacArthur Foundation, "A New Textiles Economy: Redesigning Fashion's Future" (Cowes: Ellen MacArthur Foundation, 2017), 20–21.

18. Global Fashion Agenda, "Pulse of the Fashion Industry" (Copenhagen: Global Fashion Agenda and The Boston Consulting Group, 2017), 13.

WELL-BEING: MIND AND SOUL

19. Daniel Goleman and Richard J. Davidson, *Altered Traits: Science Reveals How Meditations Changes Your Mind, Brain, and Body* (New York: Avery, 2017), 207.

20. Ibid., 249.

21. Ira Hyman, PhD, "Don't Think about It: Thought Suppression Causes Behavior Rebound," *Pyschology Today* online, September 10, 2010.

DAILY SLOW-LIVING RITUALS

22. Tiu De Haan, "Why We Still Need Ritual," YouTube, 2016.